THE

BACK PAIN

HANDBOOK

Francine St George

The Back Pain Handbook

This edition published by The Physiotherapy, Posture and Fitness Clinic, Sydney Australia
+612 9399 7399 www.physioposturefitness.com enquiries@physiopfc.com

First published 2016

ISBN 978-0-9875430-1-1

eISBN 978-0-9875430-2-8

Illustrations: Ruth Conwell

Book Composition and Layout: Sylvia Xanthos Design

Cover design: XOUM Publishing

Printed and bound in Australia by McPherson's Printing Group, Maryborough, Victoria

Disclaimer

Francine St George recommends that any person who considers they have a back condition, that is not resolving with the exercise and advice outlined in this book, must consult a medical or health practitioner.

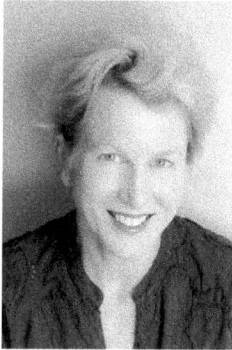

About the author

Francine St George is a Sydney-based physiotherapist who is passionate about sharing the latest research with her patients to help them overcome back pain. Francine has studied anatomy and sports science and has a Master of Science in Medicine. Her thesis topic was the correlation of Magnetic Resonance Imaging with clinical findings about back pain.

In the first phase of her career Francine travelled extensively with elite athletes as a trainer and physiotherapist. She uses this valuable experience in her daily clinical work. Francine has conducted courses for health professionals and others in her Sydney clinic, in various parts of Australia, and abroad.

Over Francine's 36 years of clinical practice, many of her patients have learned how to overcome back pain with exercise and other strategies that are covered in this book. Now it is your opportunity to learn these.

Francine practises in Sydney at the Physiotherapy Posture and Fitness Clinic. Winter or summer you will find her enjoying a swim and doing her daily exercises at one of Sydney's great beaches.

Other books by Francine St George

The Muscle Fitness Book

Simon & Schuster, Sydney, 1989

The Stretching Handbook

Simon & Schuster, Sydney, 1994, 1995

Bodyworks

ABC Publishers, Sydney, 1999

Self-published, 2002, 2007

New Bodyworks

Self-published, 2013

Acknowledgements

My greatest thanks go to my patients and radio listeners. They continually request clear and concise explanations about why their pain has not resolved. This continues to inspire me to stay up to date with the latest research and share this with them.

Much of the recent innovative research on back pain has been done by Australian physiotherapists, so thanks to my colleagues for allowing the results of their research to be available to all.

This book would not have been possible without the artistic skills of Ruth Conwell. All credit to her for transforming my outline diagrams of exercise and humour into meaningful illustrations. I'm also grateful to Mirka Kubeckova who was a model for the exercise illustrations in the book.

Sylvia Xanthos has done a great job with body composition and layout and I thank Xoum for their creativity for the final cover.

Thanks to my good friend Robyn Day and to Stephen Bennett for their editing in the early stages of manuscript development. John Carrick, as editorial adviser, helped to clarify the book, to ensure that readers could readily understand the advice and follow the exercises without difficulty, step by step.

I'm grateful to my colleagues at our physiotherapy clinic, PPFC, in particular Penny Elliott. Everyone helped with constructive feedback and provided support when I needed to devote more time to the book as it neared completion. They are a fantastic team of professionals and I really appreciate their loyal support.

Preface

In my physiotherapy practice I treat back pain every day. Fortunately, I can use advanced technology and review the current research on back pain. This knowledge is invaluable in choosing solutions for my patients.

Intriguingly, no matter how much the research has evolved over the years, these simple concepts still help to resolve back pain:

▸ you need to think a bit differently

▸ breathe a little more deeply, and

▸ keep moving.

An episode of back pain can interfere with normal daily functioning. Advances in technology have shown why this is, and also what you need to do to avert recurrent episodes or longstanding back pain.

I have experienced back pain. My original injury happened over 25 years ago. Although I recovered from the injury and superficial bruising, a deep ache and pain lingered in my back, hip and leg for many years. My back often became locked, and seeing myself in the mirror standing crookedly was not pretty.

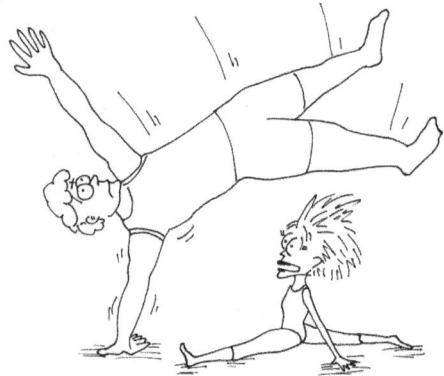

In recent years, new technologies including Magnetic Resonance Imaging and Real Time Ultrasound imaging have shown why these subsequent episodes of instability and locking occur. This information enabled me to identify the most helpful exercises and strategies for my back. I can now state confidently that you can learn these too, even if you do not have access to this advanced technology.

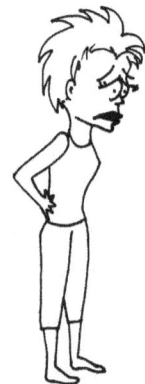

I have never labelled myself as a "back pain sufferer" nor have I thought of myself as having a "bad back". Over the years though, the pain or locking of my back has affected me physically and emotionally. Fortunately it has been some years since I have seen a crooked image of myself staring back from the mirror. It has taken diligence, commitment and investment to understand what I needed to do, but it has definitely been worth it.

Sometimes medical or surgical intervention is necessary to overcome back pain. But even if you have had or are going to have surgery, the exercises and information in this book will support the best possible outcome.

Unfortunately there is no single exercise or thought that is likely to "fix your back". But being informed of the latest research and working through the exercises and strategies in this book will help you to know what works for you and what does not. Although it is important to seek treatment as soon as possible when you are experiencing an acute episode of back pain, it is critical not to become dependent on someone "fixing" you regularly, either weekly, or year after year.

Nevertheless, if you find it challenging to understand how to do some of the exercises in this book, it is important to work with a physiotherapist or other health practitioner. They will help you to clarify which are the most suitable exercises for your back condition.

Over the years, at times, it has been a frustrating journey looking after my back, so if you are reading this book in search of solutions, I do empathise with you.

The good news is that you can overcome your back pain and lead a more normal life. From personal and professional experience, I know that it is possible.

Francine St George

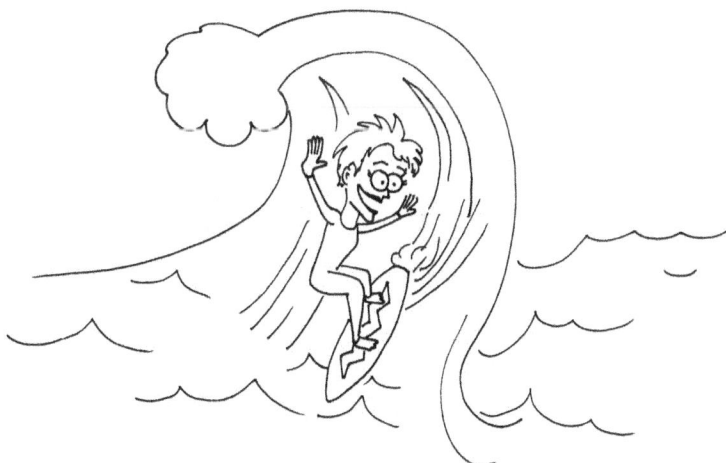

CONTENTS

1 The back pain story - breaking the cycle

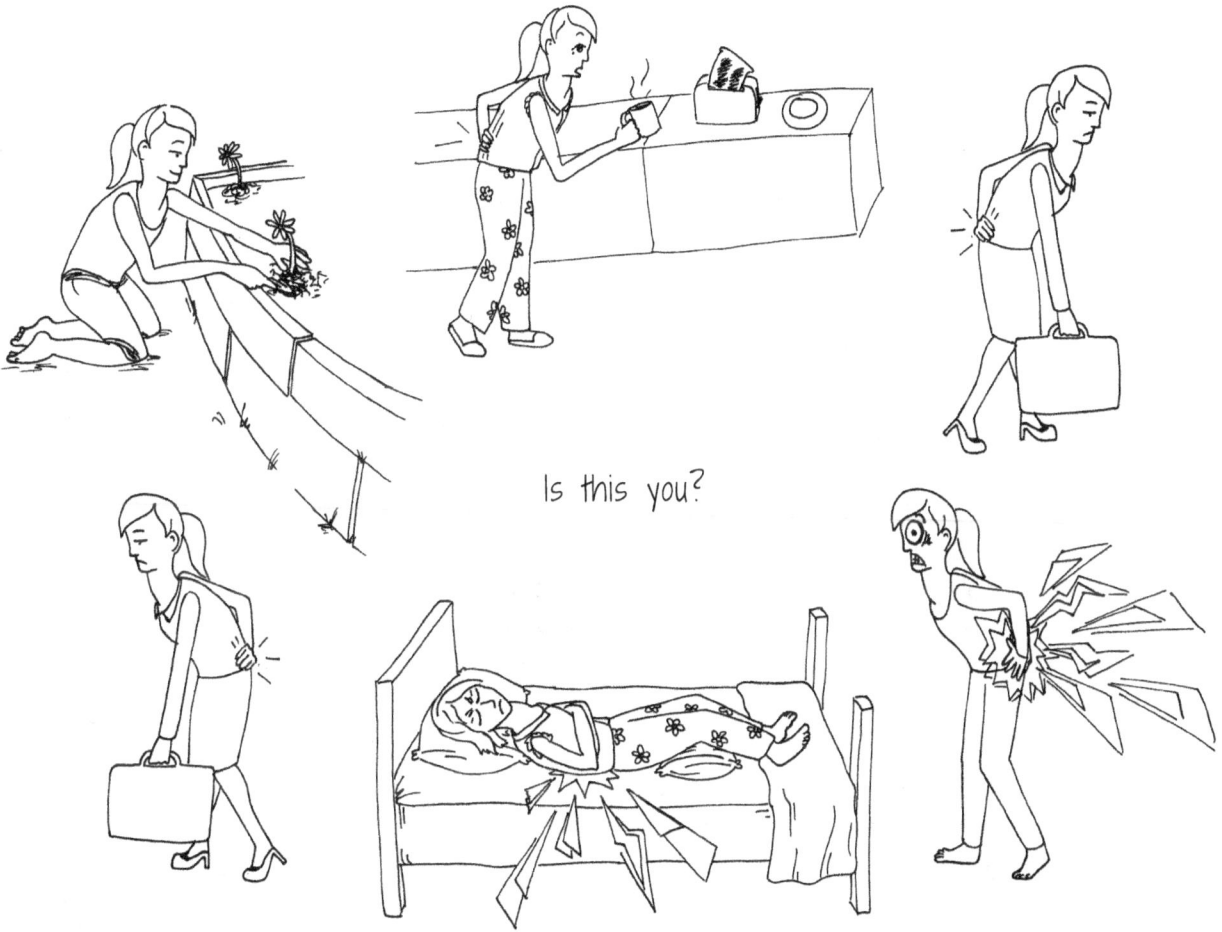

Is this you?

Figure 1. The pain cycle can start after even
one episode of back pain

There are three phases to back pain. The first phase is the onset of back pain, which might have occurred without apparent cause or through injury. You tend to ignore the incident until you notice that the pain is becoming more frequent or more intense or is taking longer to resolve.

The second phase involves seeking a cure. The pain might remain, but the process of seeking relief can be time-consuming, expensive and emotionally draining.

The third phase is putting research into action. This involves recovering from an acute episode and using early interventions to prevent the pain from recurring. My goal is to move you as quickly as possible into the third phase.

Phase 1. "The back's gone out, I don't feel so good"

When you experience back pain it is easy to think of yourself as a "back pain sufferer". However, you are not a sufferer, nor is your back "bad". When you think negatively, you move differently without realising it. You start to avoid everyday physical activities because you associate them with pain. The more you do this, the more other areas in your body start to compensate.

You may notice that when your pain is present you start to feel out of sorts or more emotional. This can make you irritable and alter how you interact with family, colleagues and friends.

These sometimes subconscious and emotional behaviours associated with back pain are now well understood. The challenge is to recognise that these things are happening and to take the correct steps, straight after your first episode of back pain. You will thereby avoid the cycle of regular treatment to overcome pain.

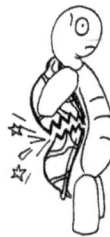

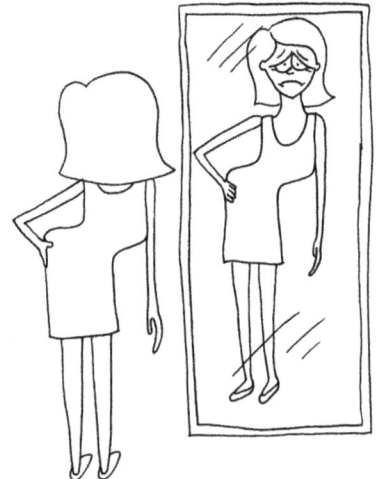

"My back is 'out';
I must have a 'bad back'"

Phase 2. Finding the help you need

Figure 2 demonstrates what most of us do when pain occurs often. Going to a general practitioner for advice on back pain is second only to visiting the doctor when suffering from a flu or cold. During their lives, 80 per cent of people will consult a doctor about back pain.

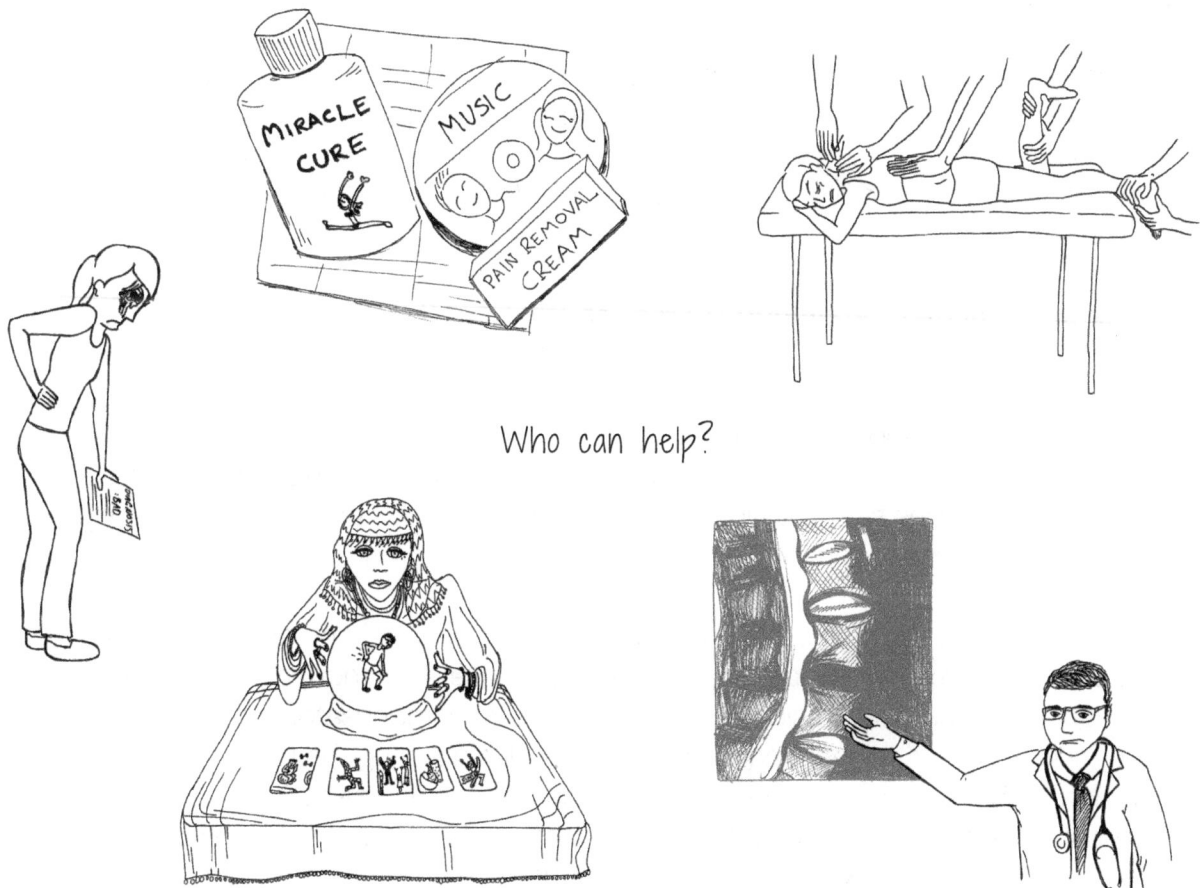

Who can help?

Figure 2. Chapters in the back pain story

You might be advised to take pain medication and tests such as X-rays, CT (Computerised Tomography) or MRI (Magnetic Resonance Imaging) scans. The findings might show a disc bulge, disc deterioration or another condition. Once you hear these terms, you could easily think that the findings revealed by the tests are the source of your pain, but they might not be. Intriguingly, the research shows that you can have a disc with anatomical changes accompanied by a lot of pain, but you can also have these changes and experience no pain.

However, once you see the results of such scans, you could easily start thinking that there is something seriously wrong. Unconsciously, you might start to limit your physical activity. Then the endless search begins as you try various treatments and fads. You might continue to hear many different terms along the way: your back is out; your pelvis is misaligned; even that you have "the worst misalignment I have ever seen," and so on. It is disillusioning when you try yet another series of treatments and at the completion the pain is still there. Often it seems simpler to just give up and accept the inevitable. You can mistakenly think that you have to live with the pain, whereas you can take steps to help yourself.

Phase 3. Recovering by putting research into action

Studies show that from the first episode of back pain, the body responds with a fight-or-flight response. This is to protect you from doing the same action or movement that caused your pain in the first place. As part of this fight-or-flight response, muscles seize up, you breathe a little differently, think a little differently, and change the way you move.

Technology can show how the brain records these physical and emotional effects. However, chronic pain can develop because even though the initial pain in your back has gone, residual muscle weakness, compensatory habits and negative thoughts might remain. The brain is still registering the need to protect you from the perceived danger of hurting yourself again, when this is no longer required. That is why you might inadvertently tighten muscles or feel emotional when you think of making a movement that used to be painful. Research has shown how to deal with the physical, emotional and compensatory habits that remain from an episode of back pain. This is essential to preventing chronic pain from developing.

Recovery...

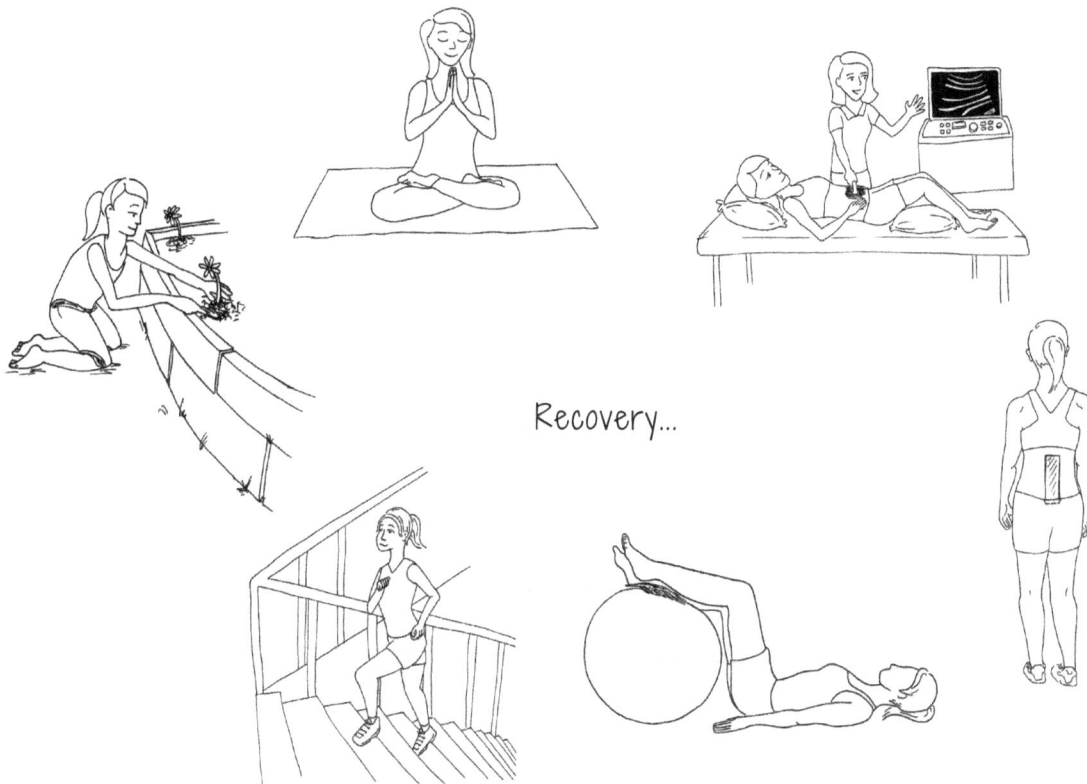

Figure 3. Seeking recovery from back pain

In the following chapters you will learn what to do if you experience an acute episode of back pain. You will be able to identify which muscles have been weakened by the episode and how to strengthen them. You will also learn which muscles compensate and become tight and how to stretch or relax them.

Changing how you react to an episode of back pain can avert the development of a chronic condition. The goal is to move into and through the third phase confidently and competently, and not stay stuck in the first or second phases.

HOW TO USE THIS BOOK

Please do not stop at merely reading about what you should be doing. Try the exercises and strategies. This will give you the best chance of having a healthy back again.

My suggestion is that you begin by reading the first few chapters on anatomy and nerves so that you have an overview of the possible causes of your back pain.

If you have longstanding pain you may have heard many diagnostic terms over the years. If so, I recommend that you read Chapter 10 before starting any of the exercises.

There are six chapters of exercises: for your back; for finding your core; and for all areas of your body. Try working through one of these chapters each week and note the exercises that feel most beneficial for you. These will be the ones that help you to move more freely or that ease your pain.

By the time you reach the last chapter, you will be able to choose a daily routine from Appendix 11 or design your own program and refer to it as you exercise.

Self-assessment

I strongly recommend that you complete the self-assessment in Appendix 1. This will record where you are now and allow you to put some helpful strategies into action immediately. I have also left spaces for you to make notes at the end of each chapter.

At the end of six weeks you will be ready to complete your follow-up assessment. You will quickly determine how you have progressed and you will be able to identify any aspects that you still need to work on.

Eventually, for future twinges of back pain, you will not need the self-assessment. You will be able to quickly and easily put into action all of the new exercises and strategies you have learned.

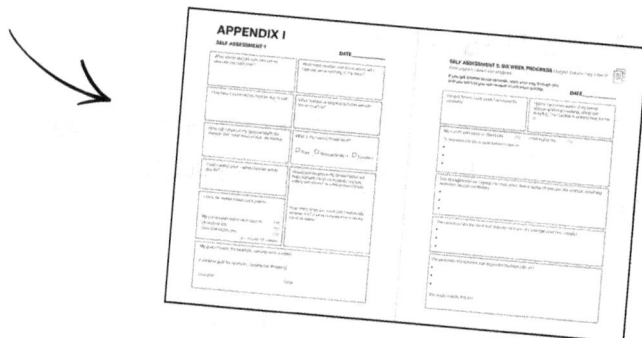

Is this book suitable for me?

The book has been written for anybody who is interested in an active, exercise-based approach to resolving their back pain. You can benefit from this approach if:

▶ your back feels vulnerable when you lift a light weight

▶ you have ever experienced a locked back

▶ you wake up feeling stiff in your lower back each morning

▶ your back aches when you sit or stand for extended periods

▶ your posture could be better

▶ you have ever sustained a back injury, or

▶ you are frustrated by recurrent episodes of back pain, despite trying many approaches.

⚠ **CAUTION:** Please consult a medical practitioner before trying the solutions offered in this book if you experience any of the following:

▶ constant night pain in either the lower back, hip or legs

▶ loss of bowel or bladder function

▶ constant pins and needles, numbness in your leg or obvious muscle weakness, for example foot drop

▶ pain that does not resolve with a course of anti-inflammatory pills or pain medication

▶ recent surgery, or

▶ rheumatoid arthritis.

💡 Questions to ask

▶ What terms do you use to describe your pain? How could you change them?

▶ How could you avoid making decisions based on how your back is feeling?

▶ When does your back pain happen? Are there some poor postural habits you could change immediately?

▶ Could you improve your overall fitness?

▶ Is it time to assess your nutrition and diet? Should you consult a nutritionist or dietician?

☰ Actions to take

▶ Do not simply read this book; do the exercises. Note which ones feel good and which ones do not.

▶ If you are not clear on an exercise, postural tip or strategy, consult a physiotherapist or other health professional who treats back pain, to learn how to apply this information to your condition.

"It's time to change things - I know I can"

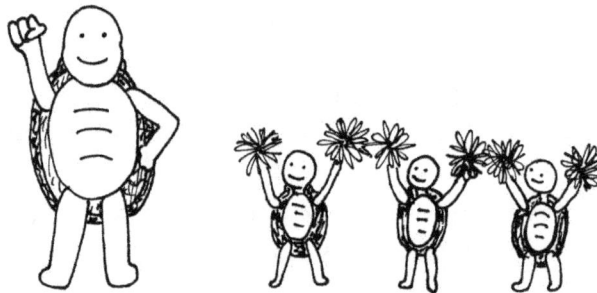

✏️ **Notes**

2 Anatomy overview

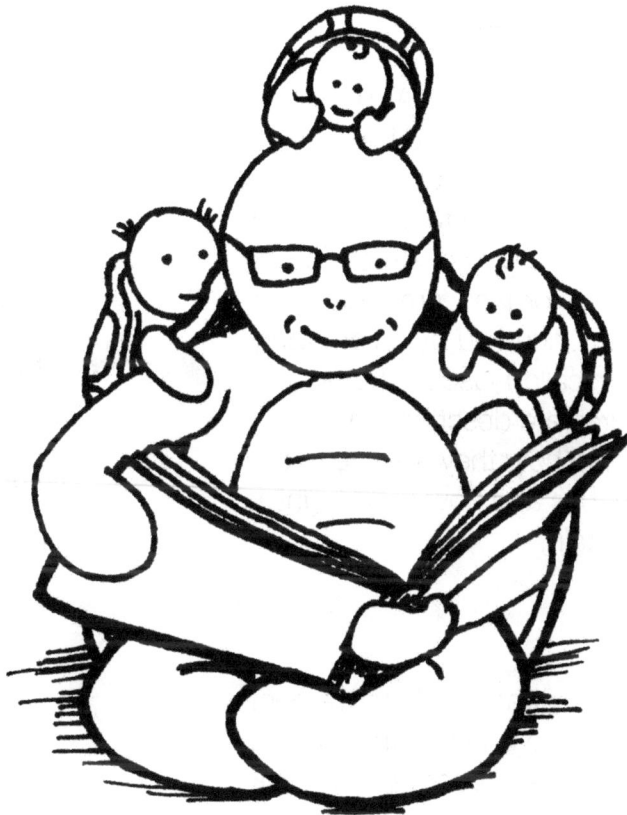

"Ok kids - story time. We're going to study just enough anatomy so that we know how pain and all our daily postural habits affect our muscles, tendons and ligaments"

Bones, ligaments and muscles

There are 226 bones in the body. All bones are held together at differently shaped joints by ligaments, which provide stability and flexibility. There are 450 muscles, joined to the bones by tendons. All of these anatomical structures, as well as our nerves and organs, are supported, separated and interconnected by an amazing soft-tissue structure called fascia. These anatomical structures are described in more detail below, outlining how they are affected by daily postural habits and how they might contribute to back pain.

The spine

There are 24 vertebrae that enable movement from the top of the spine down to the sacrum, and lastly to the tailbone or coccyx. The neck vertebrae are called cervical, the mid back thoracic, and the lower back the lumbar region. In between each vertebra is a gelatinous (jelly-like) disc that provides protection for the spinal cord. The discs, and the facet joints that are also between each vertebra, give the spine flexibility and stability. Spinal nerves exit from the spinal cord between each vertebra; as they run into legs and arms they are called peripheral nerves. Overcoming back pain requires attention to all levels of the spine.

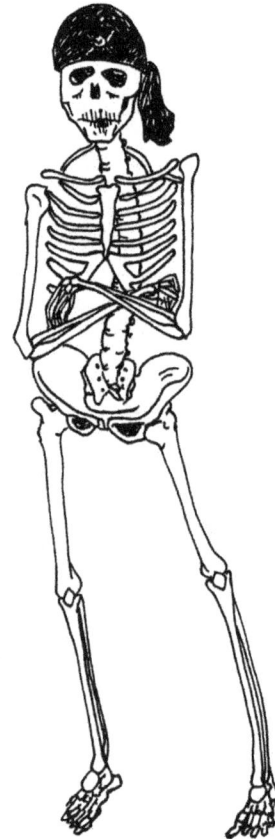

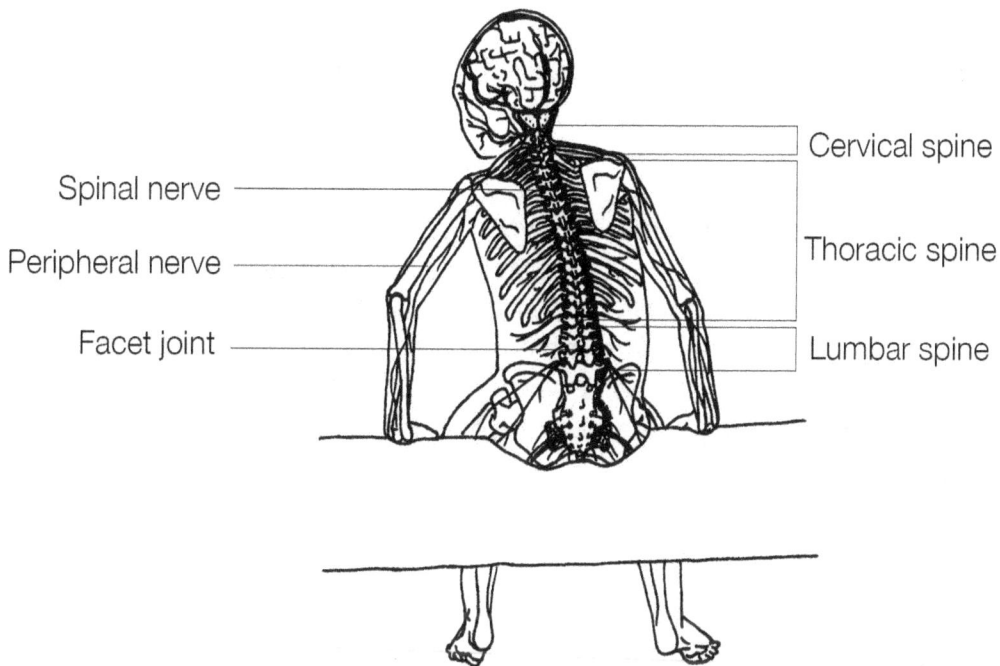

Figure 4. There are 24 vertebra in the spine. Between each level, facet joints and a disc provide flexibility and stability. Spinal nerves exit from between each pair of vertebrae and extend to all peripheral areas in the body

Muscles

Some muscles have an important role in supporting posture. Other muscles contribute more to movement.

All throughout the body muscles have slightly different functions. The main role of postural or stability muscles is to reinforce ligaments and stabilise joints. These muscles tend to be deeper and not visible to us. They have a higher content of slow-twitch fibres and are designed for endurance. They are generally working automatically, without conscious direction. For instance, you are not thinking about contracting your neck muscles to hold your head up while you are reading now. This is due in part to your stability muscles being automatically engaged.

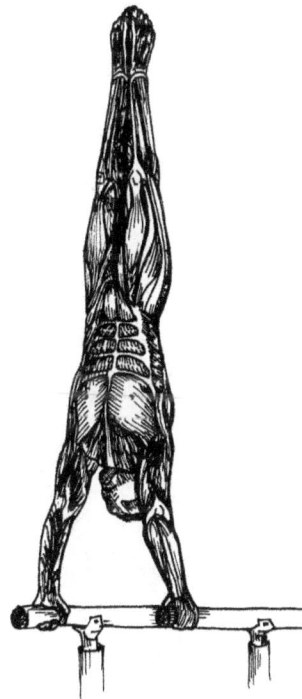

When in a sedentary state, for instance sleeping or sitting, many postural muscles are synchronised with breathing. This is important to remember when you start to retrain these muscles, which I explain further in subsequent chapters.

Phasic muscles are those that more actively involved in larger movements. When you anticipate or think about moving, stability muscles engage to stabilise joints before activation of the more superficial phasic muscles occurs. Phasic muscles are larger, longer and have more fast-twitch than slow-twitch fibres. Phasic muscles also have variable fast-twitch fibres in them and this enables them to adapt to the varying paces we move at, including walking, jogging or sprinting.

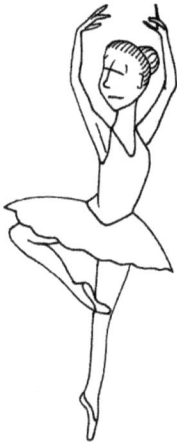

The muscles that assist poise, balance and posture are called postural or stability muscles. These are usually deeper in the body and not as visible. When these are weak in the back or hips you could tire if you stand or sit for a long time.

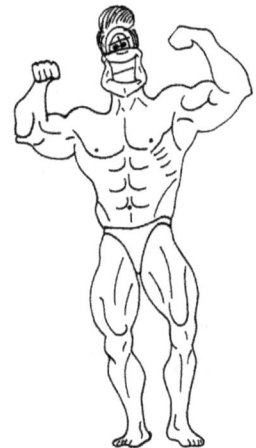

The muscles evident on the outside are for faster movements. These are called phasic or power muscles.

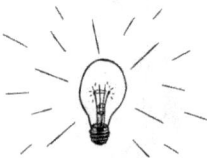

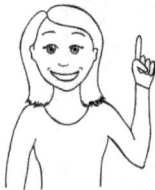

When pain occurs anywhere in the body, the deep postural muscles become inhibited. This means that they are somewhat inactive. In the back this compromises the stability of the spine.

The phasic muscles activate too quickly when you are in pain and even think about moving. This can be triggered by the smallest activity, such as bending to put on your shoes or leaning forward to brush your teeth.

The fast triggering of the phasic muscles can cause the back to lock. The deep stability muscles do not automatically activate to support the spine and the phasic muscles go into protective spasm. You will feel this as tight muscles in your back.

A helpful analogy is to compare the different muscles to the gears of a car. When you have pain and even think about moving, the body needs to jump straight from neutral (where everything is relaxed) into second, third or even fourth gear. A specific vertebral level is not able to adjust to your moving quickly, and the back may lock.

Probably one of the most important things that technology has permitted us to confirm is which specific stability muscles have become inhibited by pain and which phasic muscles have compensated. The resulting imbalance of muscles can occur at any joint following an injury. This instability might be experienced as locking but you could also experience unpredictable clicking. This is common in the hip or shoulder as well as in the lower back.

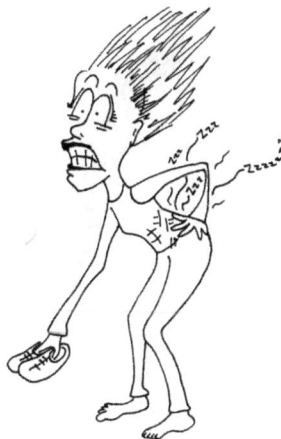

"Ah ha! So this is why my back goes out
when I am not even lifting anything heavy"

Muscles of the spine

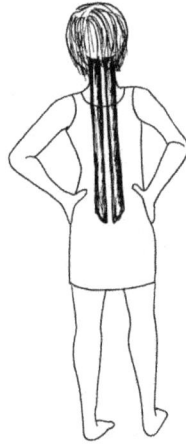

"I feel like I have two rods in my back when I have back pain"

When you have back pain it can often feel like you have two rods of muscles either side of your spine. The superficial phasic muscle group that feels so tight is called the erector spinae. It runs from the base of the spine and inserts at varying places all the way up and down your spine including your ribs and neck. If there is tightness or muscle spasm of the erector spinae, it usually indicates weakness of the deeper stability muscles.

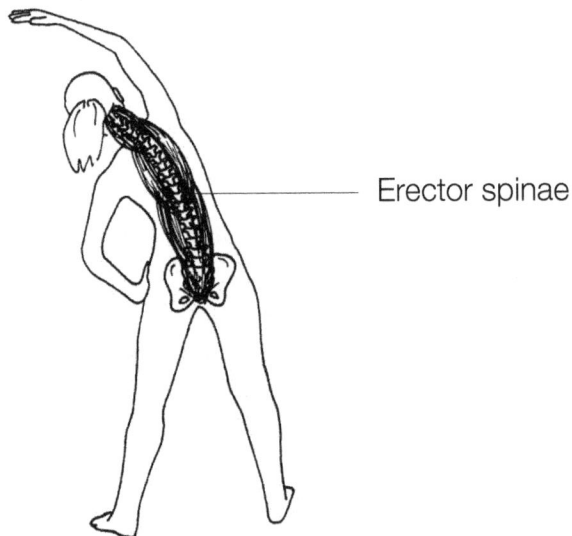

Erector spinae

Figure 5. The erector spinae refers to muscles that are superficial and have a predominantly phasic action

Underneath the erector spinae is the multifidus. This muscle has segments of various length; some run between each other; others attach to a vertebra a few levels above or below. The multifidus runs all the way from the lower back right through to the neck.

There are many other muscles that arise from the back and go to the arms and legs.

The first step in overcoming back pain is to stretch and relax the outer erector spinae and other phasic muscles that are tight, and then activate and wake up the deeper muscles that have been inhibited by pain.

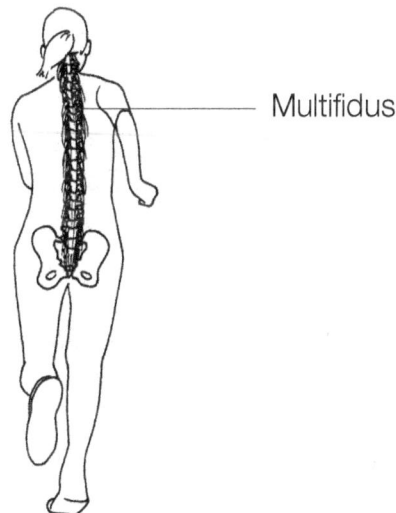

——— Multifidus

Figure 6. The multifidus is the deepest muscle of the spine. It runs between each vertebra and between a few levels of the spine

The core muscles

Research confirms precisely which muscles are compromised by back pain.

The deep muscles that contribute directly to the stability of the spine are the diaphragm, the pelvic floor muscles and the transverse abdominus. In combination with the multifidus, these muscles are often referred to as our inner core.

Any or all of these muscles can become "sleepy" or inhibited after even one episode of back pain.

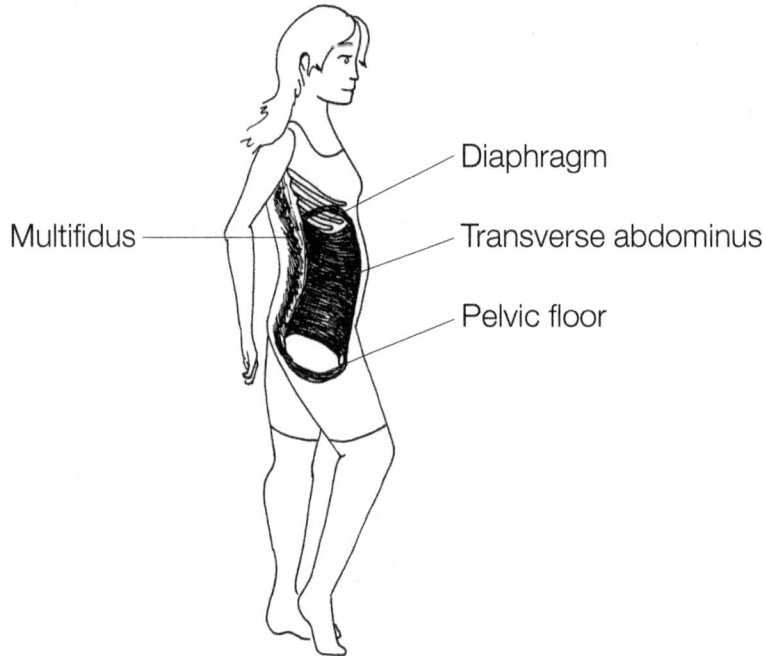

Figure 7: The muscles that comprise our inner core are affected by back pain

Because understanding these muscles is one of the most important things you need to know to resolve your back pain, they are covered in detail in subsequent chapters.

Gluteal and hip muscles

The muscles of the hips and legs have a direct influence on the back.

There are muscles at the front, side and rear that all influence stability and movement of the hips. At the rear, the superficial muscle is called gluteus maximus. Some of the deep muscles underneath include the piriformis, quadratus femoris, gluteus medius and gluteus minimus.

Daily postural habits can have a marked influence on the strength of our deep hip and gluteal muscles. Weakness of any of these muscles can cause back ache, hip pain or both. A pain deep in the gluteals can also be due to tight hip muscles; usually this tightness is in the piriformis. The good news is that correcting some of our daily postural habits, which we are often unaware of, can quite quickly provide relief from back or hip pain.

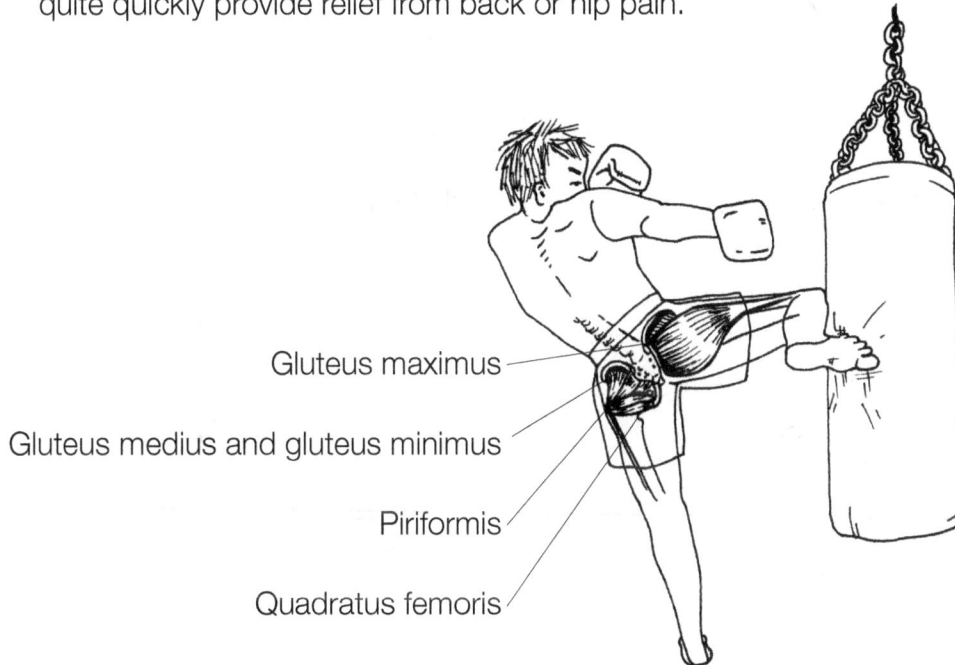

Gluteus maximus

Gluteus medius and gluteus minimus

Piriformis

Quadratus femoris

Figure 8. Important hip muscles that can cause or be affected by back pain

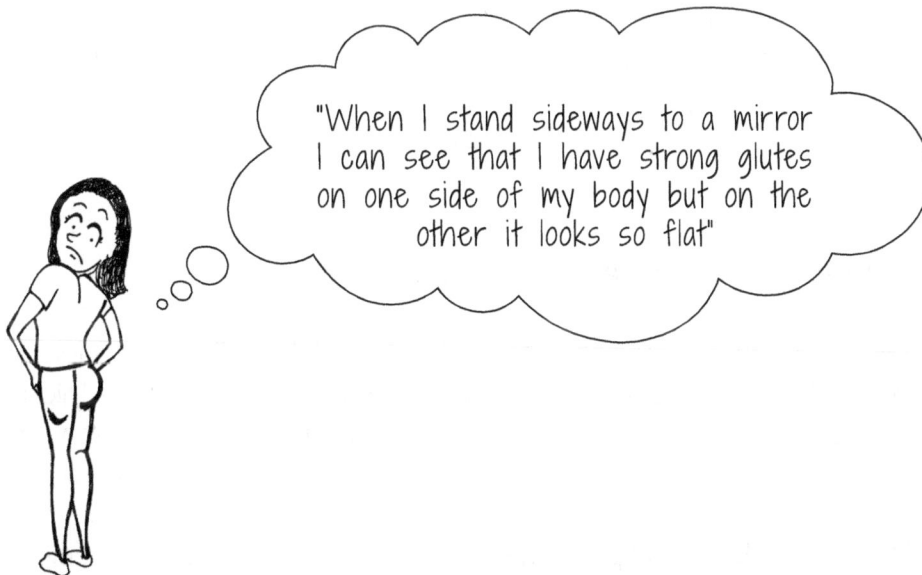

"When I stand sideways to a mirror I can see that I have strong glutes on one side of my body but on the other it looks so flat"

Postural habits could be influencing the strength of your hip muscles.

Having uneven gluteal muscles is often caused by the poor postural habit of standing with all your weight on one leg.

The first step is to try to stand on both legs evenly. The next is to strengthen the deep hip stability muscles and also the superficial gluteals. This can quickly balance gluteal strength and take pressure off the lower back.

Do you have other postural habits that might need attention?

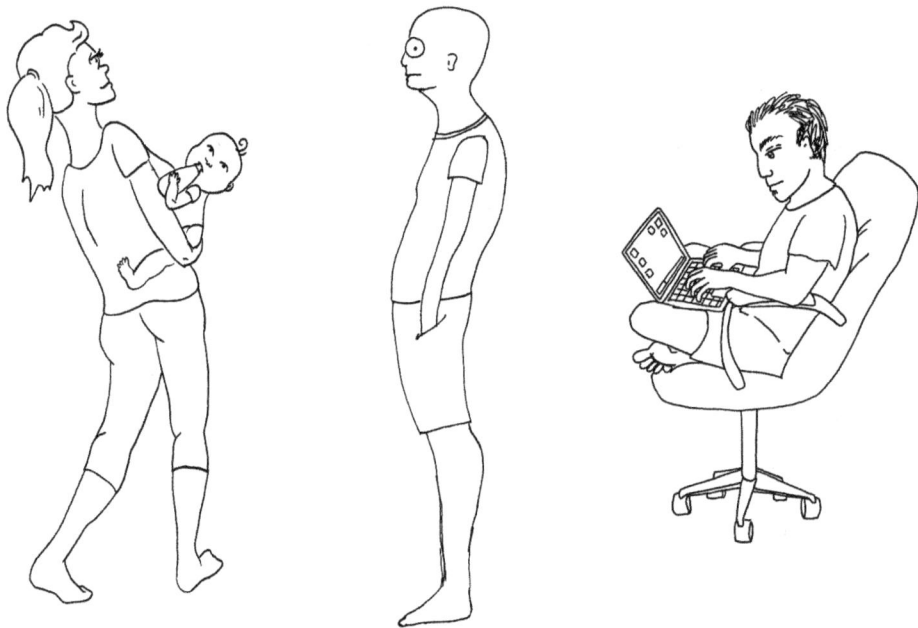

Hip flexors, hamstrings, adductors and calves

The other muscles that are important to know and that affect our back directly are: the hip flexors, iliopsoas and rectus femoris, at the front of the thigh; the hamstrings and calves at the back of the leg; and the adductors along the inner thigh. Iliopsoas is a deep hip muscle but, depending on your posture and how you habitually stand, it may be either tight or weak. Posture is covered in more detail in Chapter 9. If you spend many hours sitting, all of these muscles and muscle groups are often tight.

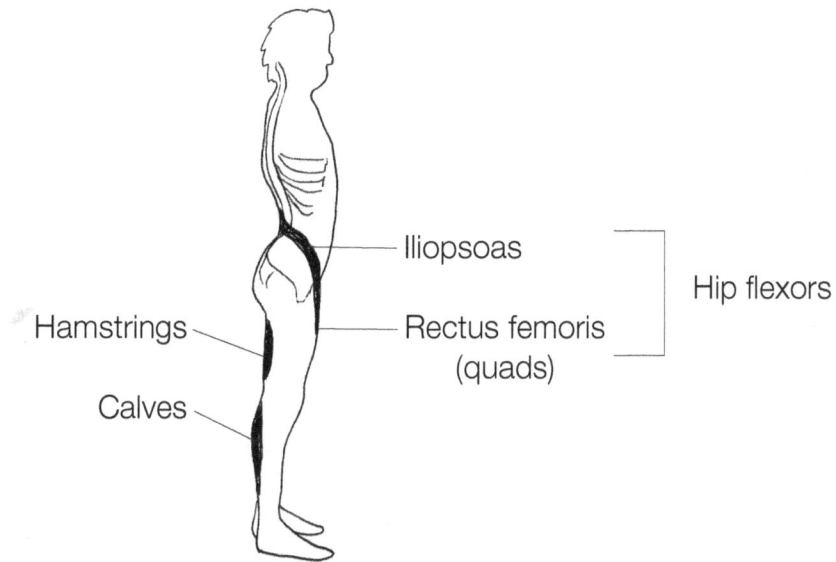

Figure 9. The superficial or larger muscle groups that are usually tight when stability muscles of the hip or lower back are weak are the iliopsoas, quadriceps, adductors, hamstrings and calves

Attention to all parts of the body

In solving back pain, all areas of the body are important.

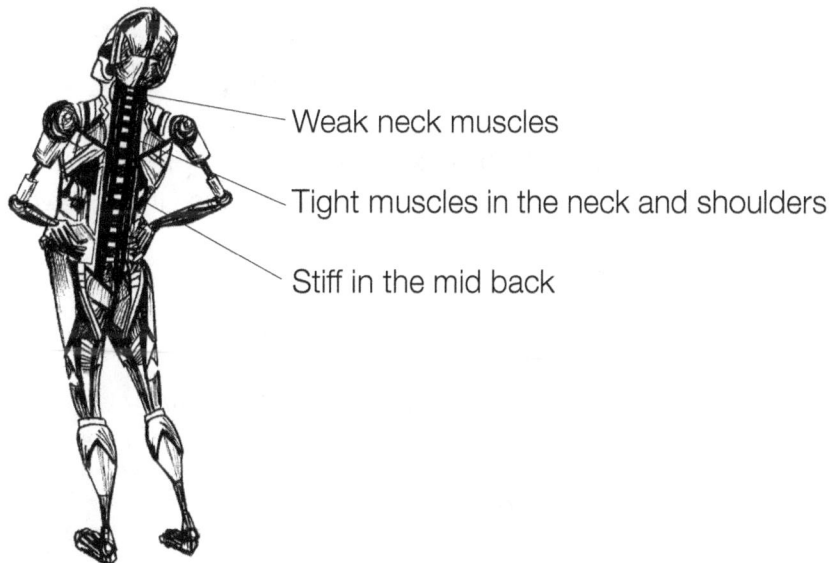

Figure 10. Some of the more common areas in the upper body that require attention

The following chapters outline exercises for the hip, legs and back as well as those for the neck, mid back and shoulders.

This information will help you determine whether any muscle imbalance in these areas is contributing to your back pain, through poor postural habits or a prior injury.

The role of tendons

Tendons attach all of our muscles to bone. However, excessive rotation of a tendon in the legs could cause a local problem such as knee or Achilles pain and also prevent the muscles of the back and hips from working efficiently. This in turn could cause back pain or hip pain.

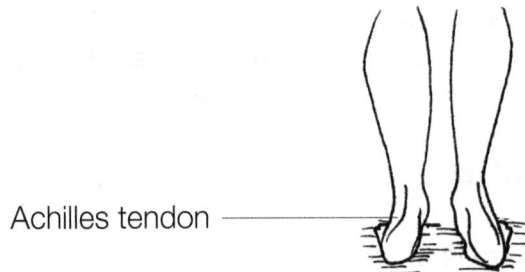

Achilles tendon ——————

Figure 11. The Achilles tendon needs optimum postural alignment for the muscles in our legs, hip and back to work efficiently

Doing stability and balance exercises could improve your postural alignment, but you might also need to consider using orthotics if you have flat feet.

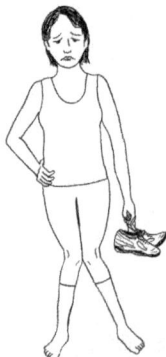

"I really want to run, but my back aches afterwards when I do. I am so knock-kneed and my feet are so flat - maybe it is time to check this out?"

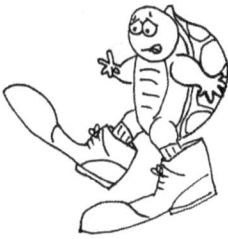

"I wonder whether I would move any faster if I used orthotics?"

Postural alignment and stability test

Try this exercise to test your postural alignment and stability.

▸ Stand facing a mirror. Now stand on your left leg.

▸ Observe your left foot – is it wobbling, and are you needing to clench with your toes?

▸ Can you see the arch of your left foot collapse?

▸ Were you able to maintain your left knee in alignment over your foot or does it roll inwards? (Checking the direction your kneecap is facing can help you decide this.)

▸ Repeat on your right leg and notice whether the foot, knee and hip alignment is different on that side.

▸ Now shift your focus a little higher to your pelvis. Repeat the exercise of standing on each leg but this time observe whether you drop laterally into one hip. It is normal to have a shift to the side, but this should not be excessive and should not cause your foot to wobble or your knee to roll in.

▸ Next, close your eyes for one to two seconds only. Please be close to a wall if you know that you do not have good balance. How stable do you feel?

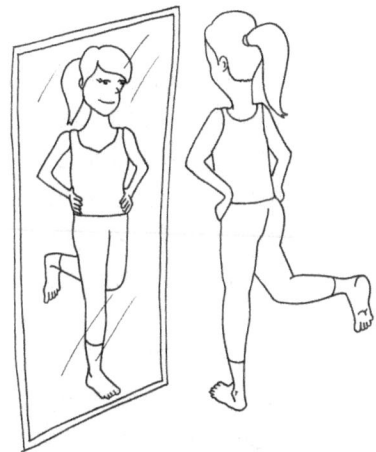

Checking your balance

Poor balance is often an indicator that you have weak stability muscles.

Ideally you should be able to stand on one leg, maintain a slight arch in the foot, not clench with your toes and not move sideways too much. Your inability to do this could be one of the factors contributing to your poor postural habits and to your back pain.

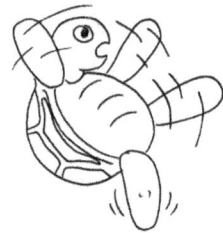

How to improve balance and postural stability

▸ Become more aware of standing with your weight evenly balanced over each foot; do not stand with all your weight on one leg.

▸ Keep your arch raised just a little as though there was a small grape under your foot and you do not want to crush it. Be sure not to claw your toes. (If you have a high arch, a less common condition called a supinated foot, lifting the arch would not be suitable for you. You can still benefit from all of the other posture tips, but you will need to relax the arch of your foot as you do each of these; do not lift it.)

▸ Move as though you were going to turn your feet and thighs slightly outwards, but minimally, so that someone who was next to you would not notice.

▸ Imagine that you are stacking all the bones in your body in a balanced way on top of each other.

▸ Once you feel more balanced in your posture, try raising each heel once or twice. Do not tense your neck and shoulders or hold your breath.

▸ If this feels too easy then tuck one foot around the other ankle and still maintain a tall but relaxed posture. This is great to do if you are at the bus-stop or need to stand in a queue for a long time.

All of these postural awareness movements and exercises will strengthen your stability muscles and improve your balance.

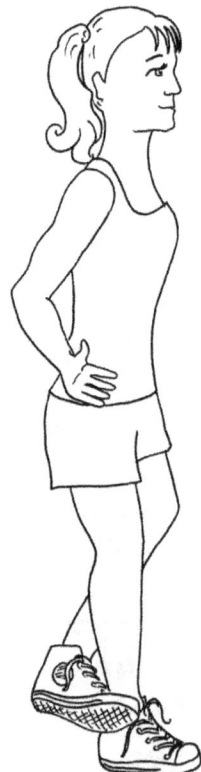

Ligaments

Poor postural habits can cause pain.

Ligaments are structures that attach bone to bone, and are similar to a new piece of elastic. They can be strained if you injure yourself or become overstretched and weakened if you stay in one position for too long.

If either a strain or overstretching occurs, the ligament becomes like an old piece of elastic. Examples of overstraining neck or back ligaments are using an electronic device in a sustained forward-flexed position, or sitting slumped in a chair watching TV. This might feel relaxing at the time but the body adapts to the awkward position. The superficial muscles in the mid and lower back and the front of the hips tighten and the deeper muscles weaken, particularly in the abdomen and core.

Can you identify a habit of being in a constantly flexed position? How could you change this right away, while you are reading this book?

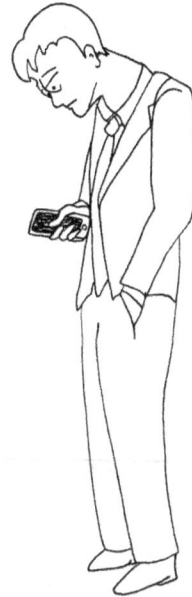

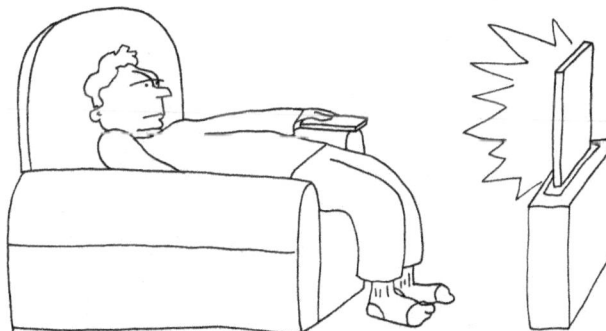

💡 Points to remember

▸ In the spine are vertebrae joined by ligaments and separated and cushioned by discs. Facet joints provide additional stability for the spine.

▸ Muscles have different functions. Stability muscles, deeper in the body, provide endurance and become "sleepy" or inhibited after an episode of pain.

▸ Superficial muscles are called phasic and have a fast-twitch function. They tend to tighten with back pain.

▸ Poor postural habits, such as standing with more weight on one leg, can create an imbalance of the muscles in the hips, which can contribute to back pain.

▸ All muscles require attention to overcome back pain, but the hamstrings, hip flexors and gluteal muscles are particularly important.

▸ Tendons join muscles to the bone. They need optimum alignment to permit ideal muscle balance in the knees, hips and lower back.

▸ Ligaments give joints stability and flexibility. If you have strained a ligament in the past or keep it in a sustained overlengthened position, muscles will adapt badly to this.

✓ Actions to take

Try the postural alignment exercise and look at your feet, knee and hip alignment in the mirror while you do it.

"Crikey - he makes it look so easy!"

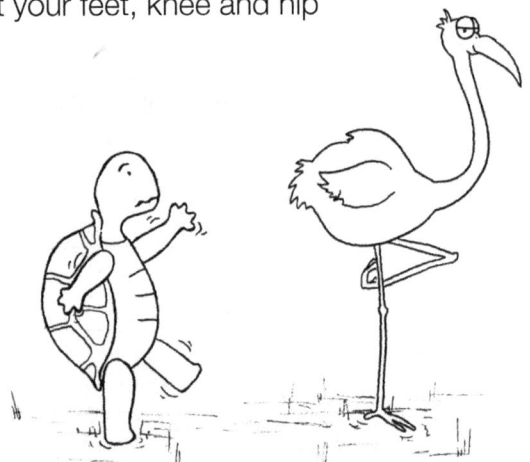

✏ **Notes**

3 Nerves and pain

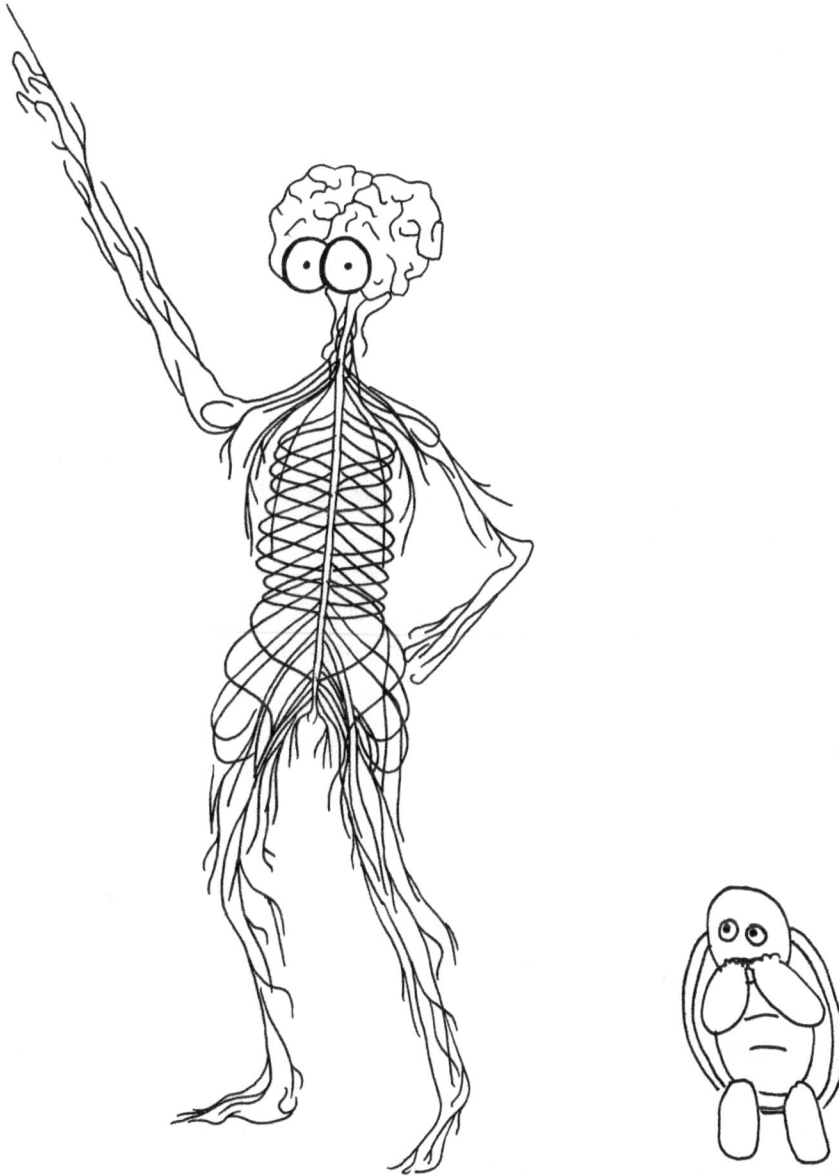

Figure 12. The continuum of nerves through the body

There might be a restriction of a nerve in its pathway from an old injury due to scar tissue or from muscle tightness that the injury caused. This could be preventing you from moving freely and confidently, even though your original injury has healed.

It is essential to do nerve exercises to help identify whether there are any other tight areas in your body (not just in your back). This might be the reason that your current pain is not resolving.

There are far too many nerves to count. The brain, spinal cord and all nerves throughout the body are well protected by strong connective tissue called fascia. When you injure yourself, nerve fascia can be damaged and become inflamed; scar tissue forms as part of the healing process. This might cause restriction of a nerve as it traverses between muscles or other anatomical structures. This is called neural tension and can cause longstanding pain to continue. Neural tension can feel like muscle tightness and can prevent you from moving freely and confidently even though your original injury has healed. Loosening a nerve in its pathway either through the spine or throughout the body is called a nerve or neural mobility exercise.

How posture affects nerves

The significant points at which the sheath of the spinal cord and its associated nerves are secured are at the top vertebra called cervical or C1 and at the tailbone or sacrum. This explains why it is so important to correct your head and neck posture so that there is no neural tension at any level of your spine. It is also the reason that a fall on the tailbone can create tension in a nerve at any level of your spine and even cause neck pain. Neural exercises can loosen any hidden areas of muscle stiffness that may still be indirectly influencing your current back pain.

Nerves have various functions

Because nerves have multiple functions in the body, your experience of pain and associated symptoms can vary. All types of nerves can create or contribute to neural tension. After you do neural exercises, your muscles can feel more relaxed; you might experience an altered sensation in an area; you might even feel quite emotional.

Here is a description of the process in more detail, focusing on nerves and the experience of pain.

Motor nerves enable the body to move; sensory nerves transmit sensation.

When you stub a toe, the brain sends messages to motor nerves to move your muscles. The pain we experience tells us not to do this again.

Sensory nerves respond to hot and cold. The body automatically responds to protect you from hurting yourself. Sensory nerves can also cause pins and needles or numbness.

Other nerves are related to our emotions and to our immune and hormonal systems.

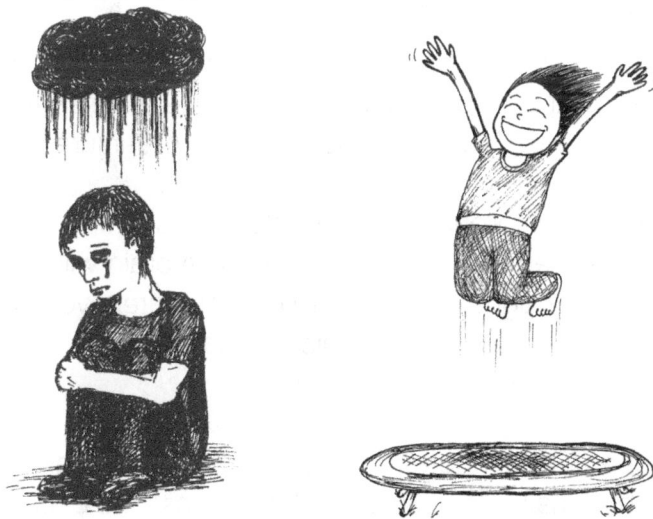

The nerves that respond to your emotions or to stress are associated with the autonomic nervous system – your protective fight-or-flight reaction. The autonomic nervous system also influences your immune and endocrine systems. The immune system fights infections and the endocrine system controls the chemicals and hormones in your body. When you are stressed or experiencing pain you can feel emotional. The fight-or-flight response remains a little overactive. The immune system can also become more sensitive with pain and you can be more vulnerable to getting a cold or the flu (the reverse is also true).

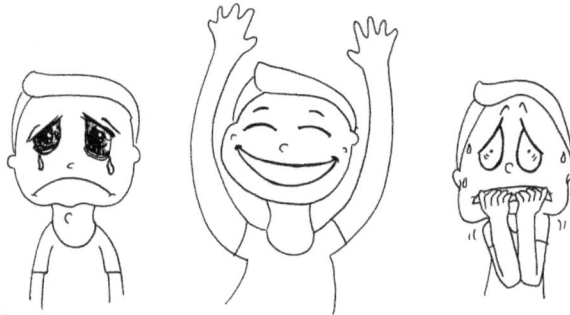

Your brain maps and responds to what is happening in the body at all times to stop you from hurting yourself.

Motor, sensory and fight-or-flight nerves are all represented or "mapped" in the brain. This is much like the GPS tracker in your car. There are also connections from the brain through the body that intersect and are filtered in the spinal cord, like the filtering of traffic at a roundabout.

There is continuous to-and-fro of messages: those from the body are sent to the brain, after filtering at the spinal cord; the brain determines the appropriate response for the body. As a result, you do not hurt or re-injure yourself.

If you are highly emotional following an episode of back pain, you will subconsciously move in an over-protective way. The brain will interpret this as needing to keep muscles tight, or in a fight-or-flight state, even when there is no longer a reason. You will experience this as ongoing pain, and you might feel tired, run down, or find concentration difficult.

The process works as if a computer program that controlled all the digitised maps in the brain had malfunctioned and all the messages became a little muddled. Technology is able to image this ongoing response to pain when an original injury or episode of back pain should have resolved. It is called brain smudging.

Nerve or pain sensors

Nerves, muscles and all other body structures have nerve sensors. These are called neurons or pain sensors. The sensors are aggravated by mechanical, chemical or sensory triggers.

Mechanical messages

If you sit on a nerve, you experience pins and needles; the brain sends a message that you should move. You do not necessarily experience this as pain. However, a tight muscle continuing to press on a nerve could cause pain, because the nerve sensors remain activated. Neural or nerve exercises, described in following chapters, can usually ease this pain.

Chemical reactions

When you sprain your ankle, there is local inflammation and swelling in the area; it is difficult to put weight on the injured leg. The brain responds; muscles go into spasm; and chemical reactions enable cells and the tissue in the area to heal. You experience pain so that you do not inadvertently re-injure this area while it is healing. The goal is to regain movement as soon as pain allows, to prevent excessive scarring in the injured area.

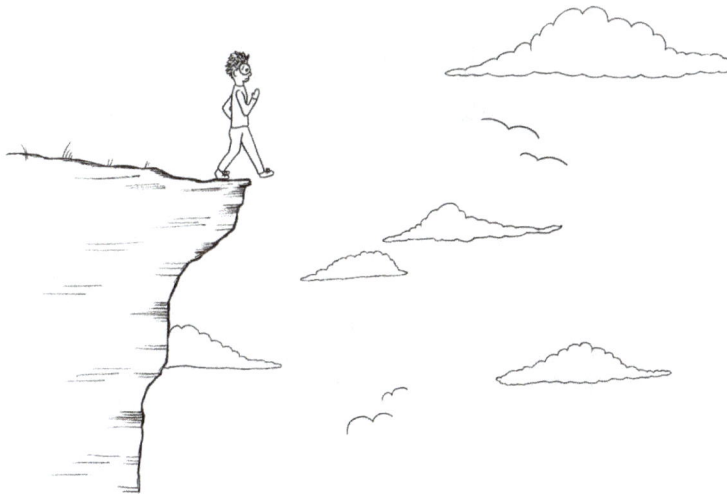

Sensory protection

Your senses of sight, hearing, taste and touch continuously provide the brain with information. This helps you not to injure yourself. In daily life, the process is mainly automatic.

Why pain can linger

Research has shown that even though a local injury has healed, nerve responses in the spinal cord or brain can still be active. This is often referred to as central sensitisation of pain. The alarm system, the nerve sensors that keep you safe, are being triggered too easily. The pain centres in the brain or spinal cord remain active when there is no longer any risk of you re-injuring yourself.

Imagine it this way: the alarm at the regional office is triggered too easily and too often. This mistakenly tells the head office that something is wrong, when the trigger was merely someone walking past the building and not even trying to get in the door.

Calming your alarm system is one of the biggest influences on how quickly you recover from an acute episode of back pain.

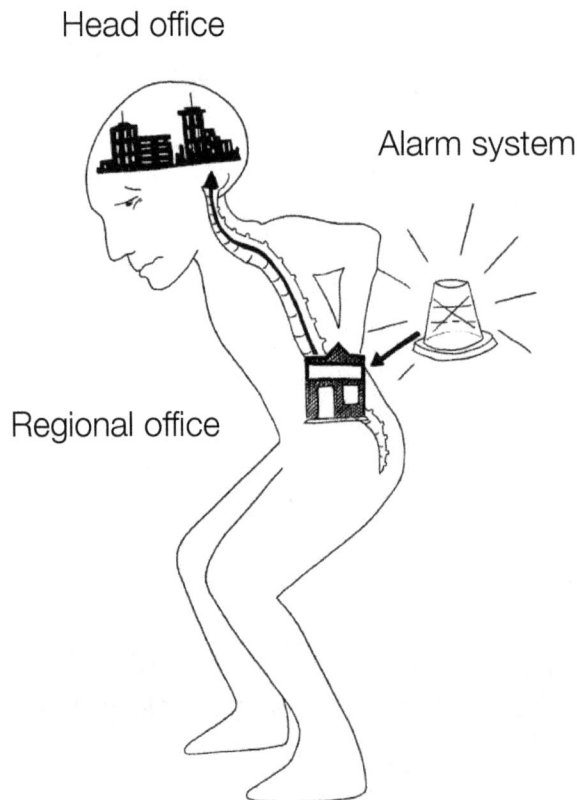

Head office

Alarm system

Regional office

Figure 13. The output from the brain depends on your reaction to pain

Activation of neurotags

Pain registers in the brain through the activation of neurotags, which are neural representations of pain.

Each individual responds uniquely to pain. The neurotags activated in your brain would be different from those activated in another person's brain. The neurotags even differ each time you experience pain.

"This pain is driving me crazy"

"I am so over having a bad back"

"It is never going to get better"

"It is ruining my life"

"I guess I've reached old age and everything will just keep getting worse"

"I've tried everything"

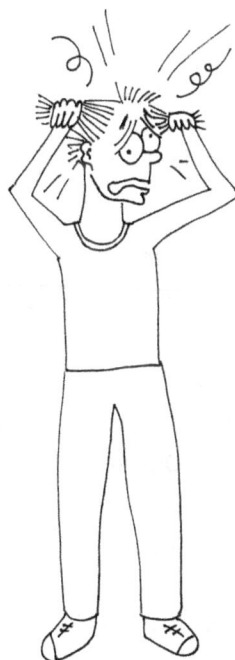

If you over-react to pain, you are keeping your alarm system activated unnecessarily. This can produce some or all of these effects:

▸ continuous heightened emotions

▸ stress through fear of having to work while in pain

▸ vulnerability to flu, because your immune system has been compromised by pain and stress, and

▸ muscle inhibition and compensatory protective habits that set in quickly.

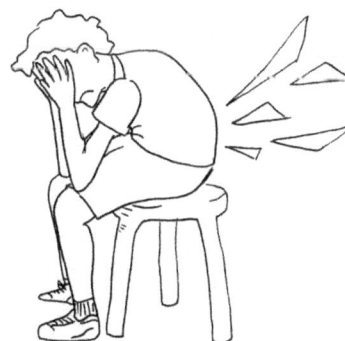

Overcoming obstacles to recovery

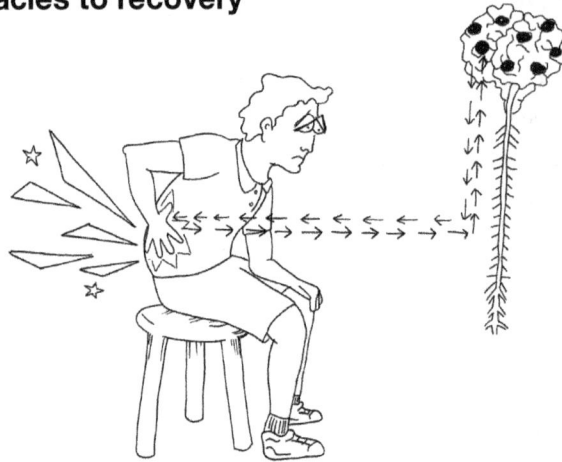

"This feels just like last time I had a bad back. It was months before I could move normally again and nobody could help me. I guess I'll just go to bed for a few days and take some pain medication until it goes away"

If you feed your neurotags with so much negative information, pain could persist for a long time. Every time you feel even a twinge of pain, all of your neurotags will respond and remain activated.

The solution is to replace your negative neurotags with positive ones.

How to recover quickly

You can move quickly through an acute episode and avoid chronic pain by starving the negative neurotags and feeding the positive ones.

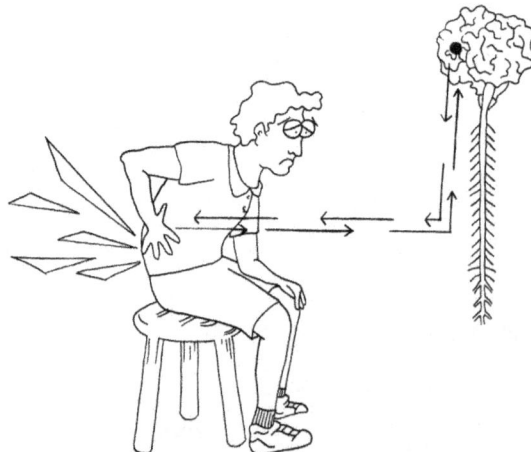

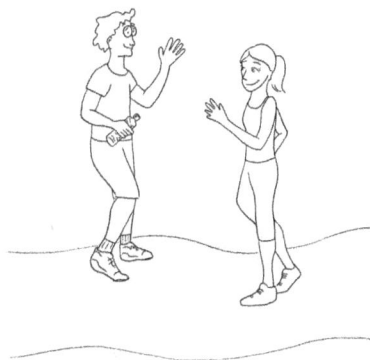

"Oh it doesn't really hurt that much. I'll go for a walk and do the exercises that I know will calm my muscles down. I will be better by tomorrow"

Calming down your alarm system will aid your recovery from back pain. As well, a positive response will help you to avoid protective postures.

By taking these steps you will experience minimal muscle inhibition, recover more quickly and avert future episodes of back pain.

Understand your reaction to pain

Being aware of your emotional response to pain is called being mindful. There are many things that influence our response to pain. Some of these include previous experiences, how our friends and family expect us to react, whether the incident occurred at work or during sport, and when we experience an episode of pain.

When you are feeling back pain, include times of calmness and deep breathing during the day. This is essential to stop your fight-or-flight system from over-reacting.

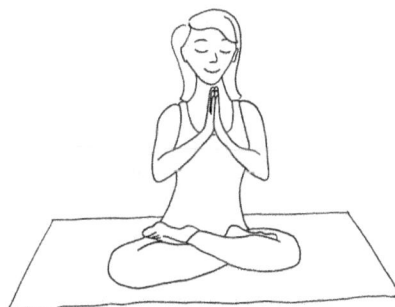

When you notice that you are feeling stressed or upset by pain, become aware of your breathing, relax your shoulders and if possible spend time by yourself until you can shift your thinking. If you can calm yourself, you will recover from an episode of pain more quickly.

Notes from the clinic

Be aware of the words you use

What words do you use to describe your back pain? What movements have you become fearful of?

When someone comes in for a consultation, I listen to how they describe their pain. I watch their emotional expression as they talk about their pain and show me what movements they fear. Often I will get the person to write down the words they are saying. They are usually unaware that they are even using these words.

Changing the words you use will help you to identify whether you are still protecting an injury when it has already healed. This is a crucial step to overcoming chronic back pain.

As you read this, take a mental note now of the words you use to describe your back pain. If the words are negative, try changing them. Think about what movements you fear in the aftermath of a previous episode of back pain. Spend a few moments now visualising yourself doing these movements freely, confidently and without pain.

Take these steps to prevent long-term back pain:

- *be aware of your physical and emotional response to pain*

- *keep fit and healthy, and*

- *move as normally as possible.*

Over-protecting the back can cause pain

A 42 year old lady, Jane (not her real name) consulted me after having eight years of low back pain and referred pain in her right leg. Jane had tried many therapies and interventions including surgery four years earlier.

Even as she told her story I saw that Jane moved tentatively and held her body rigid. Because of her long history, at the end of our first consultation I sent her away with a chart to help identify the movements and activities she feared most. I asked her to keep pain scores for sitting, for walking, and for other activities that caused discomfort.

The chart that Jane returned was revealing. Despite having a stressful job, she could sit for 8 to 10 hours with pain rated at 0 out of 10. On weekends and for movements such as dressing, swimming and playing with her children, all scores were greater than 8 out of 10.

However, her chart revealed that none of the pain she was experiencing was in her back.

At work she had no time to think about her back; therefore she felt no pain. But with all other activities she purposely tightened up her body and braced before any activity, just in case she hurt her back.

My overall impression was that Jane's back was stiff from all her over-protective movements. Over the next few months I taught her exercises to help her to move more freely. She identified more positive thought patterns and worked on improving her general health and fitness.

After some time, Jane's confidence grew and she started moving normally again. She now consults me only once every couple of months.

Jane now experiences minimal back pain, both at work and during normal daily activities.

💡 Points to remember

▸ There is a continuum of nerves throughout the body. All nerves, the spinal cord and the brain are surrounded by fascia. There can be catch points in this fascia, in the spine or anywhere in the body, from an injury. This is called neural tension.

▸ Nerves have various functions; some move muscles; some provide sensations; and others are related to the fight-or-flight (sympathetic and parasympathetic) system.

▸ All nerves have connections in the spinal cord.

▸ All motor and sensory nerves, the fight-or-flight system, and the immune and endocrine systems, have maps in the brain.

▸ If you remain too emotional and too protective of your body after an episode of back pain, all of these systems might remain over-sensitive. This could trigger an episode of pain too easily. You might simply think of a movement or activity, before moving, and your muscles could tighten up when they do not need to.

▸ To recover from back pain, be mindful of not feeding negative emotions and words to the brain. You need to respect the experience of pain and not ignore it, but you also need to focus on what you can do, not on what you cannot do.

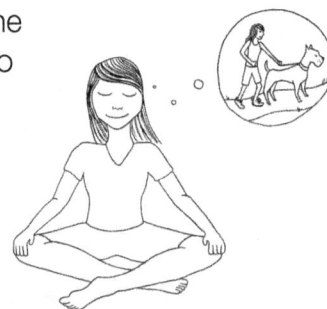

✓ Actions to take

Visualise the movements you would like to regain. If you feel stressed, focus on slowing down your breathing at regular intervals throughout the day. Try to spend some time by yourself so you able to relax a little; this will help you to calm down and not overreact to an episode of pain.

"It really is time I got off the negative thought treadmill - I know I can"

"I know this pain episode will pass"

"I will change the words I feed my brain"

"I like it that my family and friends are empathetic, but will let them know I don't want them to do everything for me. I will only develop even more overprotective habits and more pain if I keep doing this"

"I will go for a walk in the pool so that my back muscles start relaxing"

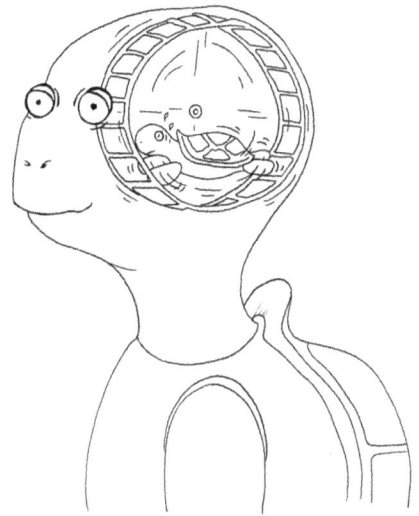

Notes

4 Neural exercises and muscle meditation

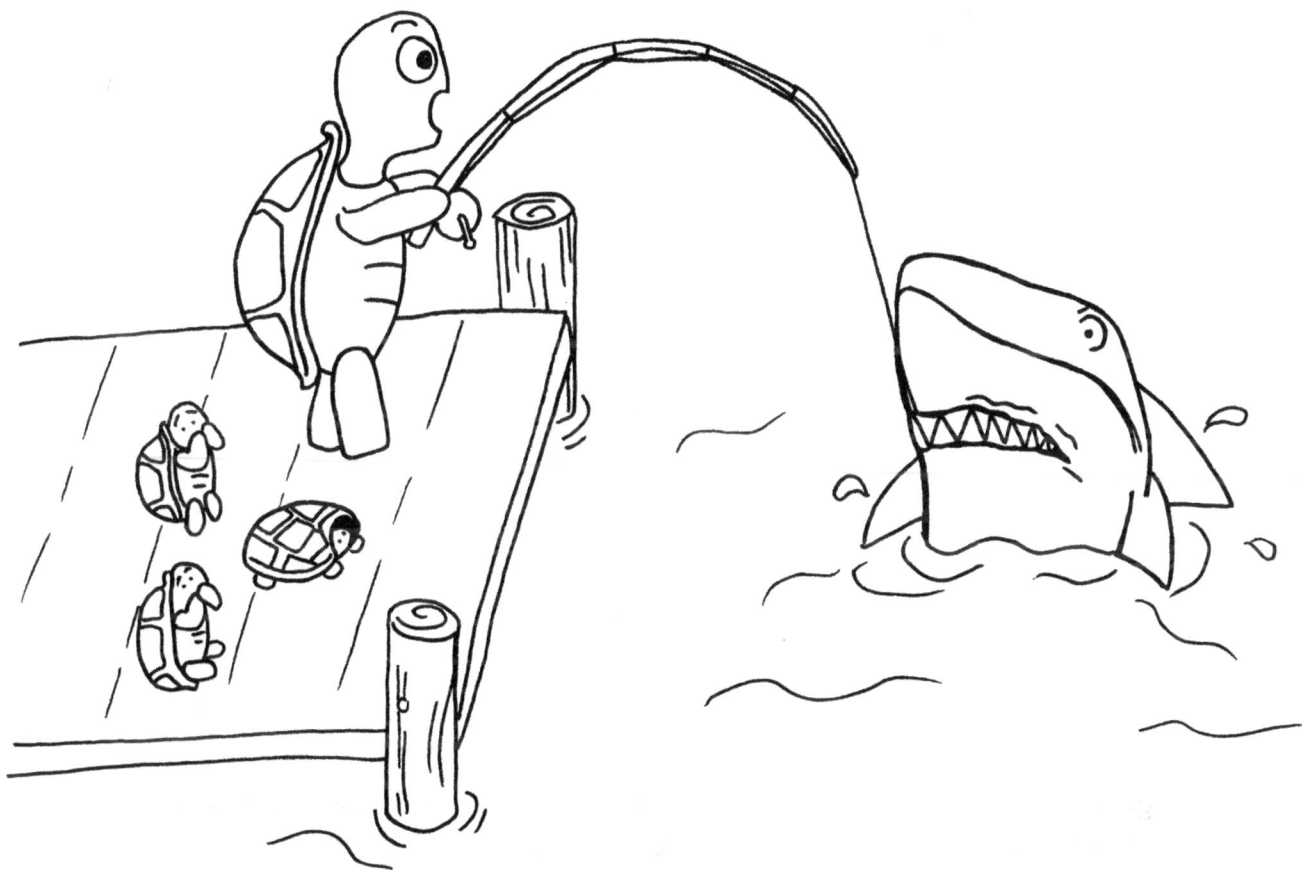

"Kids, nerves are like fishing lines, but sometimes they snag and catch on something a long way away that they are not meant to"

The aftermath of an injury that occurred many years ago, or poor postural habits might not be allowing your current back pain to settle. Neural exercises can help locate and contribute to resolving your pain. Doing neural exercises means positioning your body with the superficial muscles relaxed. Then you loosen a nerve by doing some small gentle movements with your leg, foot, arm or hand. You will also learn how to relax any superficial muscles that might be in protective spasm due to an underlying muscle weakness or because they are affected by neural tension.

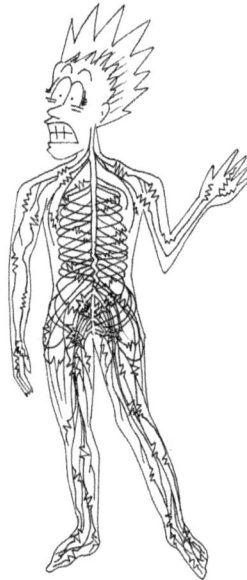

Figure 14. Nerves may have catch points anywhere in the body from a recent or earlier injury. Doing neural exercises to mobilise the nerves can release these points of restriction and enable muscles to engage and automate more efficiently. This will also help ease your pain

Be gentle with your nerve exercises

You need to be highly cautious when you start neural exercises. Nerves must not be overstretched. If you do these exercises quickly or too intensively this could increase your back pain. Overdoing them could also cause pain elsewhere in the body, where you had not known that you had muscle stiffness or tightness.

If you overstretch a nerve it will show up as a latent ache, some time later, usually about 30 minutes after you have finished the exercise. To avoid overstretching a nerve, be more gentle and reduce the intensity of the movement you are doing, but do not stop the exercise altogether. Remember to relax as many superficial muscles as you can while doing neural exercises.

Remember the original injury

It is easy to forget injuries from the past and only recall them when back pain occurs. But you need to consider old injuries to help solve longstanding back pain. Can you think of any earlier injuries now that you thought had resolved? Maybe they have not?

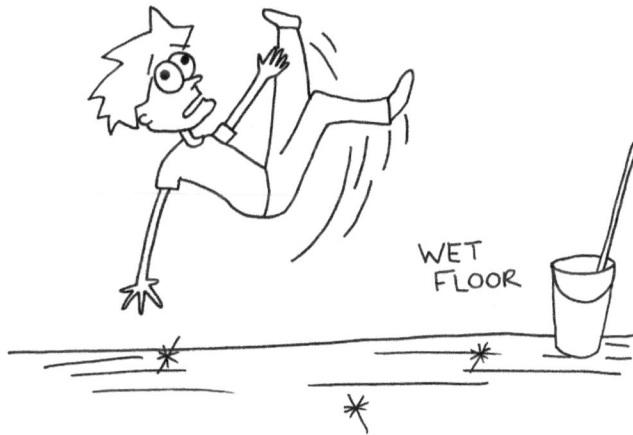

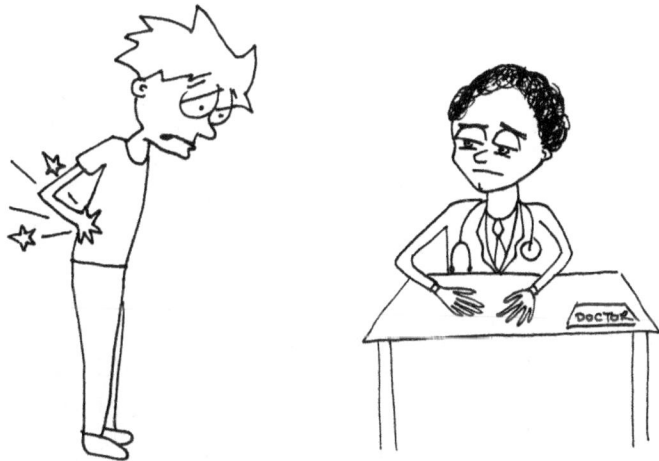

"Doc - I'm really struggling with this back pain"

MOBILITY EXERCISES WHILE SITTING

Start with neural exercises for the arms, shoulders and upper back. Do these before exercises for the lower back and legs. Even if you do not recall a previous injury, be aware that poor postural habits are often the reason for upper body tension, which could be contributing to your back pain.

Your neck and upper shoulder muscles will usually feel more relaxed after you do upper body exercises. After doing them, check whether your lower back muscles also feel a lot more relaxed. If they do, be sure to add the upper body exercises into your daily back-care routine.

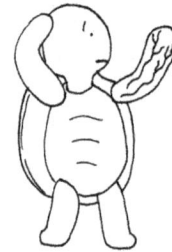

Exercise 1. Fingers facing upwards

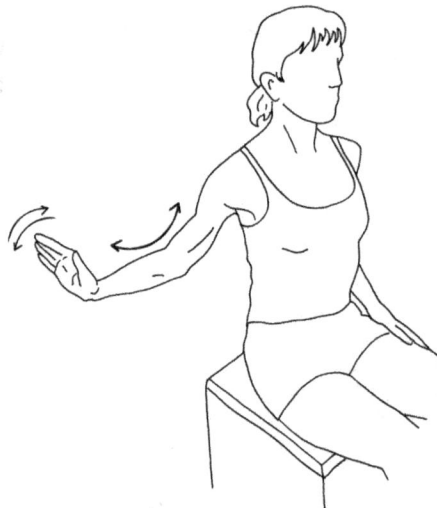

Stretch your hand out to the side of your body with your fingers facing upwards. Imagine there is a wall there and you are gently bending your elbow, just a little and almost straightening it, while moving your hand towards and away from this imaginary wall. Keep your hand at about waistline level and then start to move your arm backwards slightly behind your body. If you feel tightness in your hand, you have tension in the nerves running from your neck into your forearms. If you experience pins and needles in the hand as you do this exercise, lower your arm, decrease your wrist extension and bring the elbow a little closer to your body.

Exercise 2. Fingers facing outwards and downwards

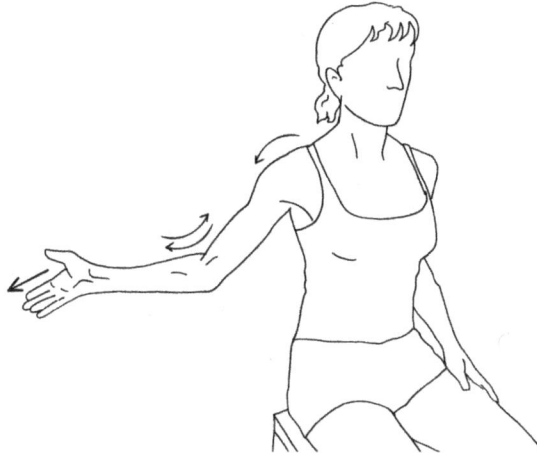

While sitting in a chair, turn your fingers downwards facing the ground with your palm still facing away from your body. Start with the elbow bent and then try to straighten it. Do this very gently with small oscillating movements. Be sure you expand the chest and pull the shoulders back and downwards for the exercise to be more effective. Again if you experience an uncomfortable pins and needles sensation in your fingers, then lower your arm, lessen the angle of the wrist extension and bring your elbow closer to your body.

Exercises 1 and 2 are highly effective in easing neck, shoulder or forearm muscle tightness, particularly if you are working for extended hours at the computer. You can also easily do them sitting or standing.

⚠ **CAUTION:** Do not stretch your arm outwards too quickly when you are doing neural exercises. If you get pins and needles in your fingers you are overdoing it. Be gentle, and be sure to correct your neck and back posture before you start moving your hand and arm backwards.

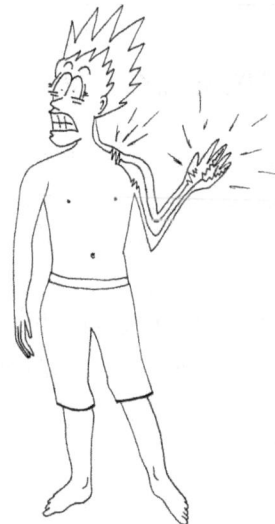

Take this test of nerves

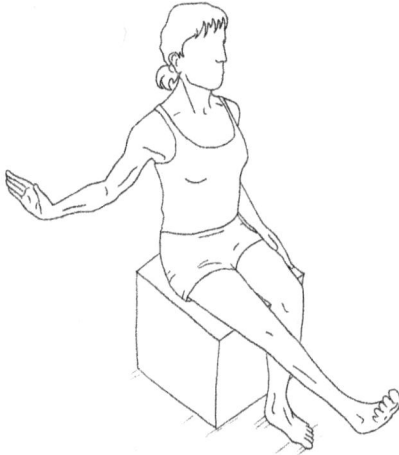

This exercise will test whether a restriction of the nerves in your neck, mid back or shoulders is contributing to your back pain.

As you do either of the nerve exercises for your arms, try this: extend your leg, straighten your knee and pull your toes back towards you. Does this create more nerve sensation in the forearm, or do you find you cannot take your arm quite so far behind you?

If you feel more tension in your arm or fingers when you extend your leg, this could mean that the tightness in your neck and shoulders is contributing to your back pain (and of course vice-versa).

Now do the following nerve exercises for the lower back, hips and legs. Then repeat the sitting arm neural exercise and extend the leg. If your arm feels looser with your leg extended, you know that doing nerve exercises for your arms and legs is essential for solving your back pain.

NEURAL EXERCISES FOR THE LOWER BACK, HIPS AND LEGS

Please be careful. None of these exercises should cause pain. If you feel tight in your leg or foot simply ease the tension off the stretch position and work more gently. The goal is to be able to have minimal tension in your back, hamstring or calf muscles while your hips are at 90 degrees. This is the angle your hips are in when you sit, so this is the position you need to be in, to ensure that you have no back tightness or neural tension.

Exercise 3. Nerve mobility for the back and legs

Lie on your side with both knees bent and place a pillow between your knees. For comfort, you might need another pillow under your head. If you can, place your hand behind you, on your back muscles. If your back muscles feel tight, readjust your body a little so that you can find a position in which they feel more relaxed. Usually, re-adjusting your legs backwards a little by extending your hips (that is, not having your knees as high) achieves this. If your back is still not relaxed, place a rolled-up towel under your waistline; this will usually help.

Now extend your knee, and as soon as you start to feel your back muscles tighten, flex the knee and take the leg backwards a little again. Draw the toes towards you and point the foot. Do this ankle movement four or five times. Take the top leg back to its resting position. Repeat the exercise two or three times. The goal is to have no tight sensation in either the foot or anywhere down the leg from the back to the ankle and be able to keep your hips at 90 degrees. Your back muscles should start to relax after you have done the exercise a few times.

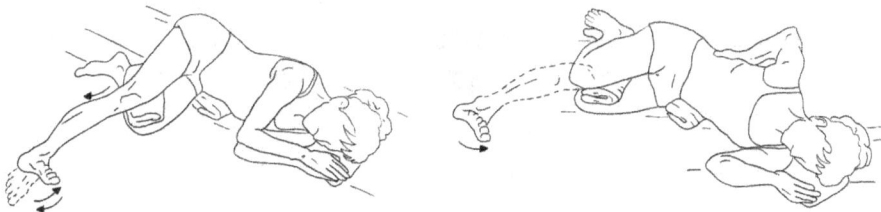

⚠ **CAUTION:** If this exercise increases the ache in your back, hip or leg, stop doing it for the time being and consult your health professional.

Exercise 4. Neck, arm and mid back, side-lying

Lying on your side, interlock your fingers and place your hands behind at the base of your neck. Place a pillow between your knees and keep your hips in a flexed position. There must be no pain or muscle tightness in your back. You may need to place your hand around and onto your back to check this first. Alter the position of your legs by not flexing at the hips as much; this should help your back muscles to relax. Now breathe in, and as you exhale, let the top arm and elbow stretch backwards. Let your head rotate as you extend your elbow. Return to the start position. Repeat this stretch three times, then rest.

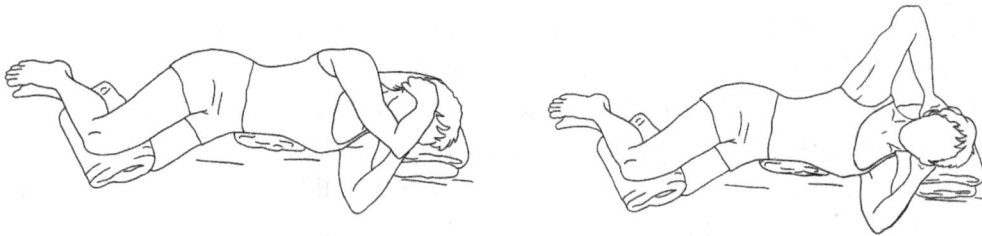

Check neck tightness

This is another exercise that will enable you to check whether tightness in your neck, shoulders and mid back is influencing your back pain.

Still lying on your side in the start position of Exercise 4, extend your leg and see whether this makes it harder to stretch your arm backwards. If it does, this may show that stiffness or nerve tension in your neck or mid back is contributing to your back pain. You will probably find Exercise 4 especially helpful for easing your lower back pain if you are experiencing an acute episode; in which case, be sure to include it as part of your daily back care routine. Remember to do this exercise on both sides, even if your back pain is on one side only.

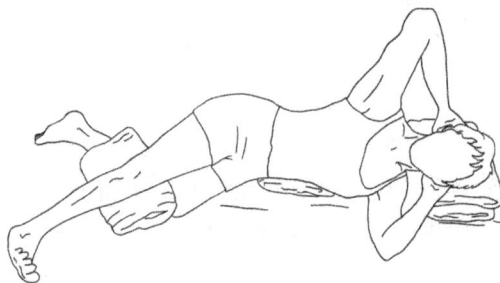

Exercise 5. Neural exercise using the wall

If you are starting to find the other neural exercises easy, and they are not increasing your back pain, it is time to progress to a more advanced neural exercise. I call this a functional nerve exercise. The intention is to loosen the nerves while the spine is in flexion (bent) and extension (straight). Be sure the exercise flows smoothly.

Stand facing a wall. Let your body fall forwards, and catch the wall with your fingers. Your weight will be on the front part of your toes. Breathe in, and as you exhale, tuck your chin in a little, and bring your knee up towards your chest. Breathe in again, and as you exhale, extend your leg behind you, ensuring that you do not hyper-extend (overarch) the back. Bend the knee twice, while your leg is behind you. Repeat only two or three times on each side.

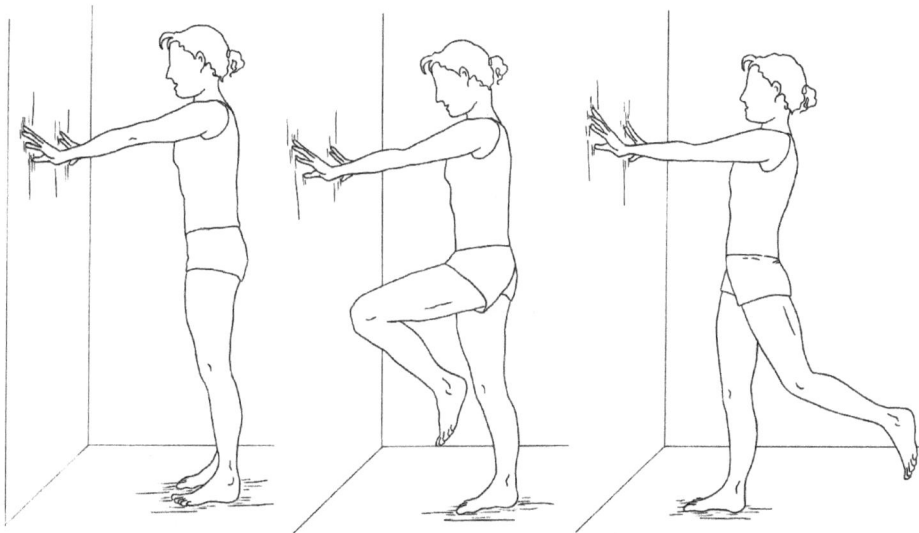

Notes from the clinic

The best exercise position to ease back pain

If you are working with a health professional who has recommended adopting a slumped posture to ease your back pain, this might be acceptable. However, if you are doing neural exercises for the first time with no professional supervision, I highly recommend that you do neural exercises while lying on your side.

Because of the anatomical connections of the fascia of the nerves that are secured at the top part of the cervical spine, it is possible to overdo this neural exercise when you flex or extend your head. This may increase your back pain.

Doing neural exercises while lying on your side enables you to monitor your back muscles and ensure that they stay totally relaxed. If you feel the muscles in your back tighten in this position, check the instructions above for Exercise 3 to learn how to prevent this from happening.

Slumped position: not recommended

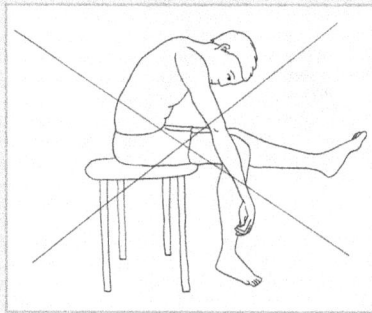

Lying on your side: recommended (Exercise 3)

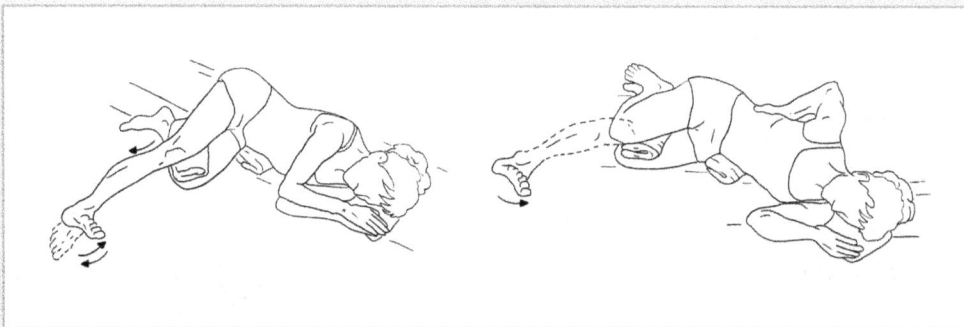

Stretching and relaxing tight muscles

For nerve mobility exercises to be effective, you need to relax or stretch the muscles that are tight because you might have been inadvertently using them to protect your back. In the lower part of your body, the muscles that are usually tight and compensating for an underlying weakness in the back and core muscles are the hip flexors, adductors and hamstrings. You may feel this as tightness at the front of the thigh where the hip flexes, or as an ache on the outside of the hip.

In the upper body, the muscles at the front of the chest and top of the shoulders are the ones that usually tighten. Much of this is due to a sedentary lifestyle. You will learn how to relax and stretch the neck and shoulder muscles in later chapters.

Stretching by itself is sometimes not enough to relax muscles that feel tight. Muscle meditation can help. It means becoming aware of a muscle or group of muscles, discovering whether they are tight, and learning how to relax them.

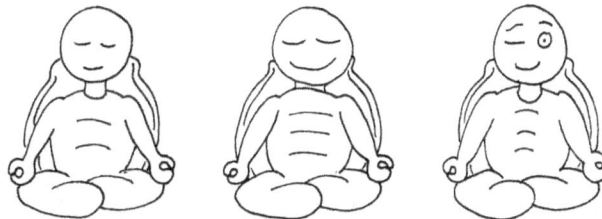

Muscle meditation can be an excellent way to ease acute back pain. Developing muscle awareness can make it much easier for you to do neural exercises.

During acute back pain you might need to relax the superficial muscles to get yourself moving a little more easily. Even if you have longstanding back pain this can be an excellent way to relax your hip flexors, hamstrings and adductors. You will find it much easier to do neural exercises and you will give your core muscles a chance to work automatically, as you move more normally.

If you have a sedentary occupation, or you drive for long periods, you will easily feel how tight the hip and leg muscles can become.

Exercise 6. Relaxing the hip flexors while supine

Lie on your back with your legs up over the seat of a chair. Place your hand on one thigh and literally pick up all the bulk of your quadriceps. How does it feel? Compare it with the other leg. If you are unsure precisely what you are feeling, place your thumb at 90 degrees to your hip flexor tendons. This is the prominent tendon at the front of your hip. It will feel like a tight rope under your fingers. Now tense and firm up one quadriceps and you will feel the tendon contract. Push your heel into the chair to tighten your quadriceps muscle. Relax this muscle, and then relax it again.

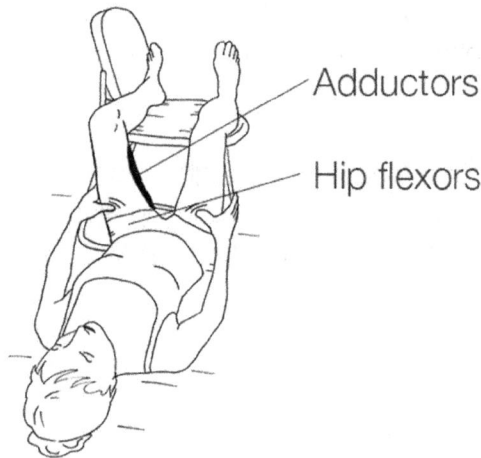

Adductors

Hip flexors

The goal is to find a position where your hip flexors are totally relaxed. You might need to drop your leg slightly out to the side to achieve this. Resting your legs up on the lounge and letting a leg rest against one end can work really well. You will need to keep readjusting the position of your pelvis and back to find the most relaxed position for your quadriceps. This is a good thing to do; it means your back muscles are starting to relax too.

Once you have done this for your quadriceps, now do the same thing with your adductors and also your hamstrings. To do this, place your hand on an adductor, the muscle on the inner thigh of each leg, tighten it and then figure out how to relax it a little more. Do the same for your hamstrings.

Relax as you work

You can relax the hip flexors when you are sitting at your desk. Do as you did when lying down. Place your hand on your quadriceps, tighten it and then relax it as much as you can. You will probably need to adjust your posture, which is a great thing, until you can relax your quadriceps totally. Do this if your back tightens after driving. But take care when doing this exercise in the car.

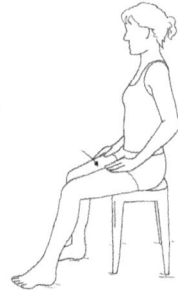

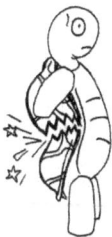

"When my back goes out I can't even contemplate getting onto my back and putting my feet over a chair. What else can I do to relax my hip flexors and calm my back muscles?"

If you cannot lie down and put your feet over a chair, the following protocol might help you to move more easily.

Exercise 7. Relaxing the hip flexors while prone

▶ Place a pillow under your abdomen; you might need someone to help you do this.

▶ Keep breathing into the diaphragm, that is, not shallow neck and shoulder breathing, and the spasm in your back muscles should start to settle.

▶ Once your pain starts to ease, push yourself onto your elbows and relax into slight extension, with the pillow under your chest instead of your abdomen.

▶ When you feel ready, raise onto your hands, but do not collapse into your lower back.

▶ Engage your abdominal muscles and if necessary support yourself on a chair as you stand up.

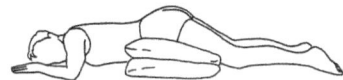

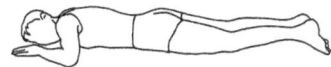

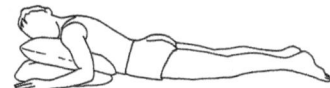

Exercise 8. Back extension while standing

▶ If you can walk and move more freely after doing Exercise 7, try this now. Place your hands on the inward curve of your lower back to support it as you gently arch backwards. Do this four or five times every few hours until you are moving normally again.

▶ Go to Chapter 5 and learn how to do postural sway to activate your core muscles.

⚠ **CAUTION:** If your back still feels locked or you experience more pain after doing either the extension protocol or the muscle meditation for your hip flexors, please stop immediately. It is vital that you consult your health professional to learn the correct procedure for an acute episode with your specific condition.

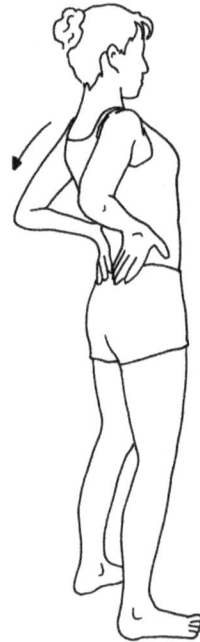

Using a brace or tape

It can help to wear a back brace or an elasticised corset for one or two days to let your back muscles settle. Take the corset off to exercise and sleep; use it during the day until you build up your confidence to move more freely again.

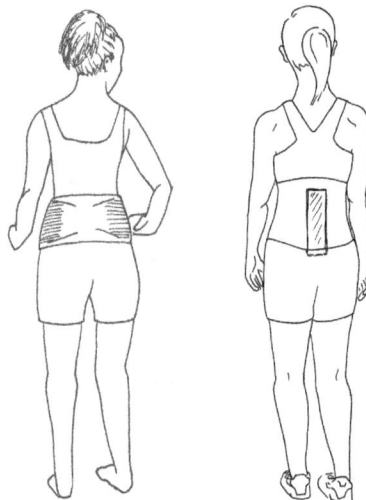

Taping can also help you through an acute episode of pain if you do not have a back brace.

To do this, place adhesive tape lengthways down your spine. This will remind you to stop bending or slumping when you sit and when you go to sleep.

This is challenging to do by yourself so I recommend that you get someone else to help you. You can leave the tape on for a few days, but the goal is to remove it as soon as your pain allows. Be careful as you remove the tape. Do not use tape at all if you have highly sensitive skin.

If your job entails heavy lifting or hard physical work and you have had pain in the past, I recommend wearing a corset as you return to work. The long-term goal is to strengthen your back muscles so that you do not need to use a corset at all.

Notes from the clinic

Wearing a back brace at times is fine

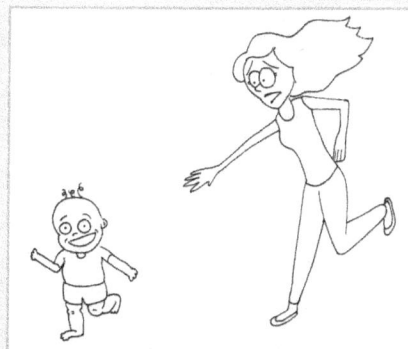

I treat a delightful lady who travels some distance to see me four times a year. When we first met a few years ago she had been experiencing recurrent episodes of locked back for over 20 years. She was aware that the pain had intensified after the difficult birth of her third child. I tested her core muscles with Real Time Ultrasound Imaging and it turned out that she had been doing her pelvic floor exercises incorrectly for many years. She was bearing down, pushing the pelvic floor muscles downwards. This would have been destabilising all the other core and back muscles. This explained the back locking episodes she had been experiencing over the years. She learned how to engage her pelvic floor muscles correctly and her back pain and associated sciatic pain settled quickly. However, she still felt vulnerable when her grandchildren were at her house and she was required to move in unpredictable ways. She felt guilty that she needed to wear her brace. However, because she had had back pain for so many years, I supported her decision to wear the brace on such occasions.

The goal is to not to depend on a brace by using it all the time. Such dependence would prevent your back muscles from returning to the healthy state they were in before you experienced back pain.

More ways to handle an acute episode of pain

Actions to avoid:

▶   Do not rest in bed for more than a few hours if you experience recurrent episodes of back pain. Bed rest will delay your immediate and long-term recovery.

▶   Do not remain in a flexed position for a long time; this will increase your pain.

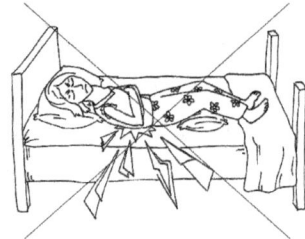

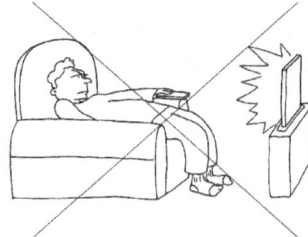

Actions to take:

Calm your muscles with ice or heat. Ice is used for inflammation and to reduce pain. If you have sustained an acute back muscle injury during sport or through lifting a heavy weight, apply ice for the first 24 hours. Be sure to place some wet material between the ice and your skin to prevent an ice burn.

Heat is preferable for recurrent and chronic back pain. One of the reasons for this recommendation is that the superficial muscles have usually gone into protective spasm. They have done that to compensate for residual muscle weakness from previous back pain episodes.

Relax the superficial muscles using some of these forms of heat:

▸   take a warm bath and add some Epsom salts or
    relaxing bath salts

▸   use a cream or adhesive plaster (available from
    a pharmacy) that provides superficial warmth to
    your muscles, or

▸   apply a heat pack (also readily available).

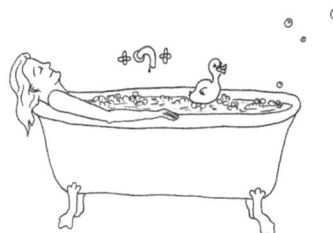

Once the muscle spasm and tightness calm down and you can move a little
more freely, restart some gentle stretching and core exercises. Your overall goal
is to move as normally as possible as soon as you can.

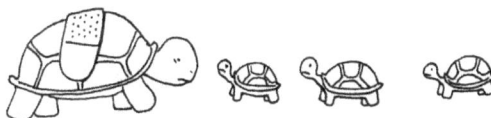

"Ok kids, let's try going for a walk"

Massage can help

A professional massage can help relax muscles in
spasm. You might find it more comfortable to put a
pillow under your abdomen while being massaged. It
is vital that heavy pressure is not applied to directly
onto the midline of your lower back. After the
massage, your back should feel more relaxed and
you should be able to start some gentle stretches
and exercises.

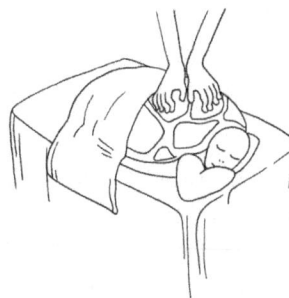

SUMMARY OF NEURAL EXERCISES AND RELAXING THE HIP FLEXORS

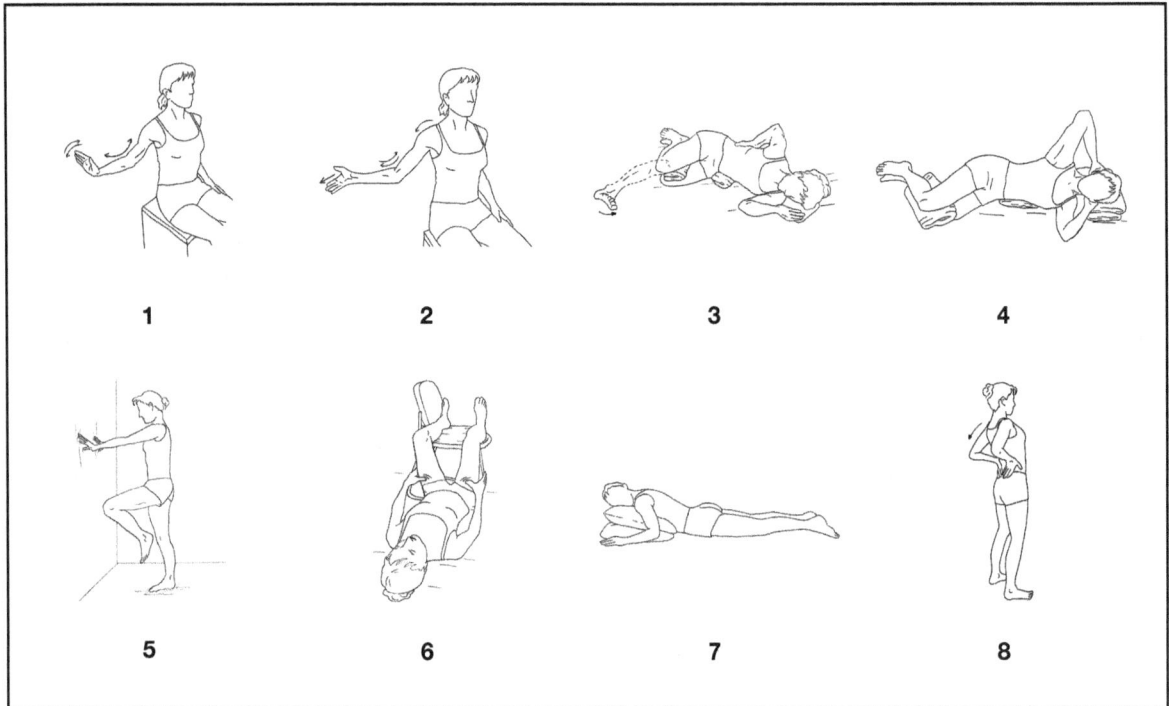

💡 **Points to remember**

▸ Some of your past injuries might have healed, but there might still be a nerve restriction somewhere other than in your lower back. Nerve mobility exercises can help you decide whether tightness in other areas of your body is a cause of your ongoing back pain.

▸ You might experience neural tension as pain, or it could feel like a tight muscle.

▸ You need to do neural mobility exercises for the upper and lower body, to relax your lower back muscles.

▸ It is critical not to over-stretch when doing neural exercises. If you feel latent pain, 20 to 30 minutes later, either in the back or somewhere else in the body, it is probably because you have been overdoing the nerve exercises. If so, you need to be more gentle, and do the exercises more slowly.

▶ In an acute episode of back pain, be careful not to overdo neural exercises. If you experience more pain after doing them, you need to stop and consult your health professional, who will advise on the appropriate exercises.

☑☰ Actions to take

You have learned various ways to relax your hip flexors, including when you are sitting for a long time. This might help you get through an acute episode of back locking. It could also help your back muscles to relax if you have had longstanding pain.

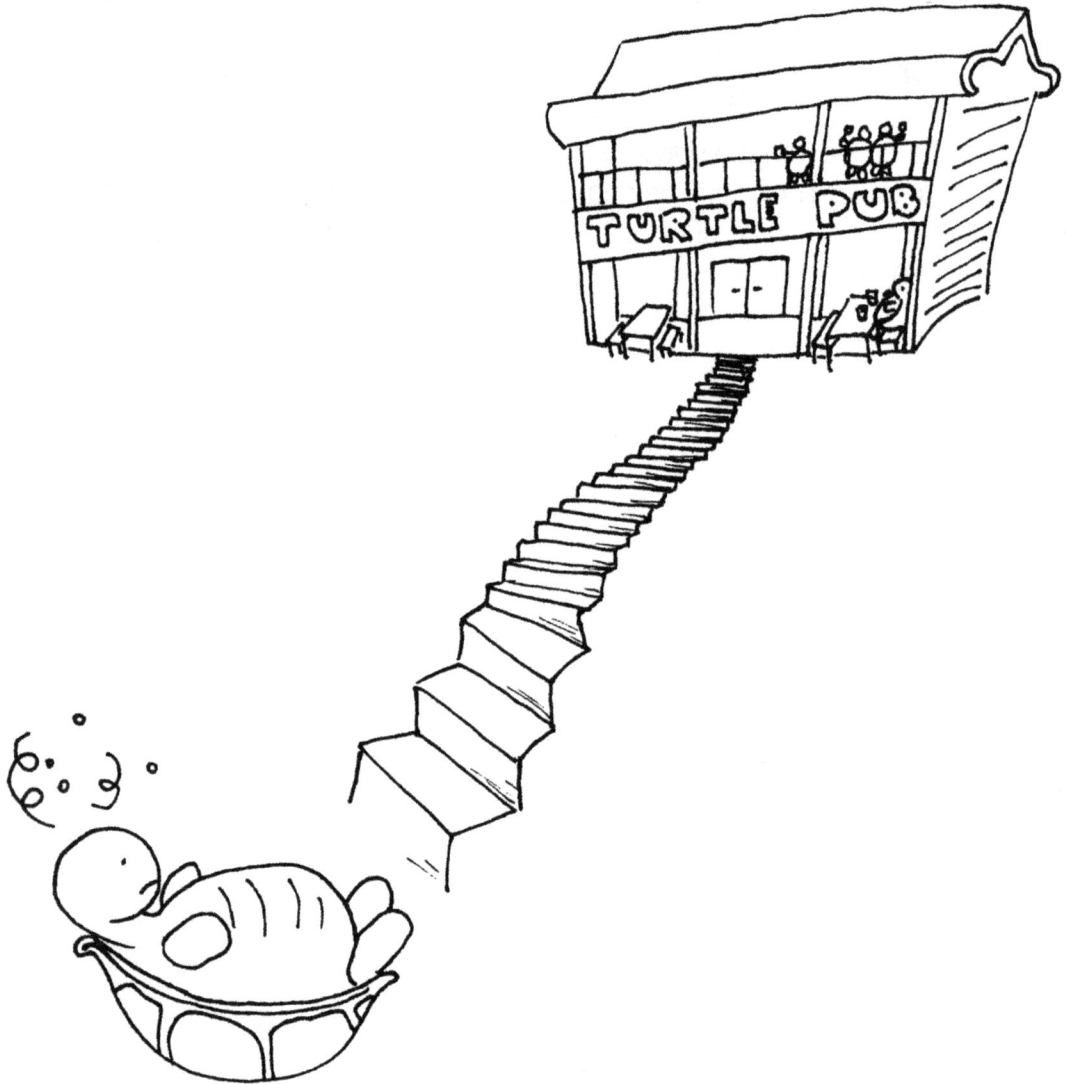

"Maybe that fall a few years ago is why my back pain is not settling? Not sure I can totally recall how I landed"

✏️ **Notes**

5 Finding the core muscles

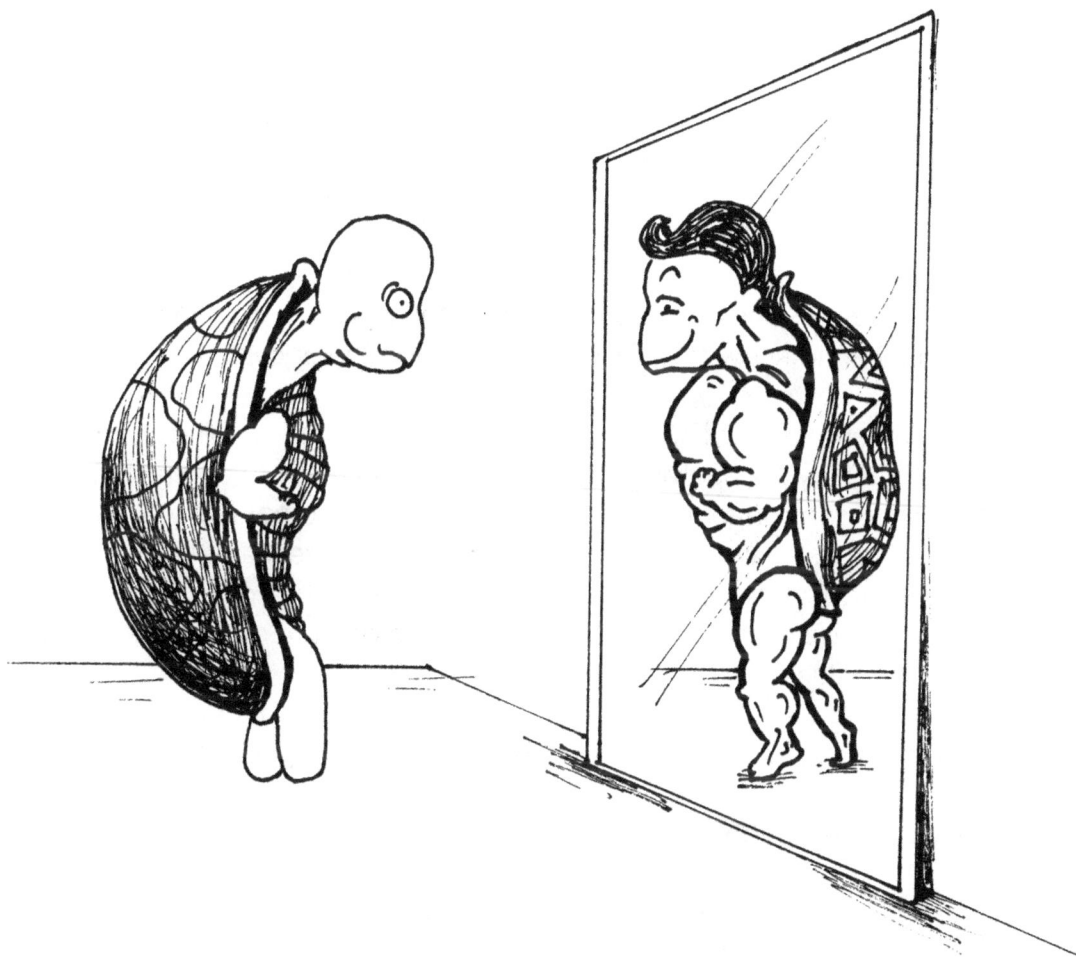

"I think I look great when I suck my tummy in and use my core muscles - but I can't breathe - maybe I'm doing something wrong"

The term "core stability" has become popular in the past few decades. It has been advocated as a cure-all for problems ranging from headaches to painful toes. Many people teach core stability in multiple ways.

Core stability alone is not the cure for back pain. However, advances in technology, including Real Time Ultrasound Imaging, now permit us to observe precisely which muscles have been affected, after even one episode of lower back pain. These include the transverse abdominus, the pelvic floor muscles, the diaphragm and the deep fibres of the multifidus muscle in the back. These are the muscles of the inner corset or core. After an episode of lower back pain, any or all of these muscles can become sleepy and inhibited. To retrain them correctly, you need to know exactly where they are in the body.

The most common problem I see, when I test how someone is doing their core exercises, is that they are applying the same level of intensity to contracting these muscles as they do for their weight training. If you do not use weights, this means the resistance that would be required for an arm wrestle or to lift a heavy item. This is overdoing the contraction required to retrain the core muscles and can increase your back pain. Once you learn how to do core exercises correctly, back pain often settles.

Below is an outline of how to locate and exercise the core muscles.

Anatomy of core stability

Figure 15 shows the key anatomical components of the corset or inner core. One way to think of your core is that there is a muscle at the top, others at the bottom and a corset of muscle that wraps around the abdomen, connected to the top and bottom muscles. Sometimes the core is described as a canister; the weakened part is affecting all other parts of the canister. This is oversimplified, but it is a good starting point.

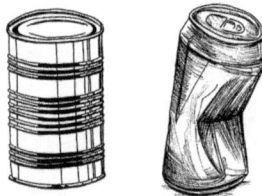

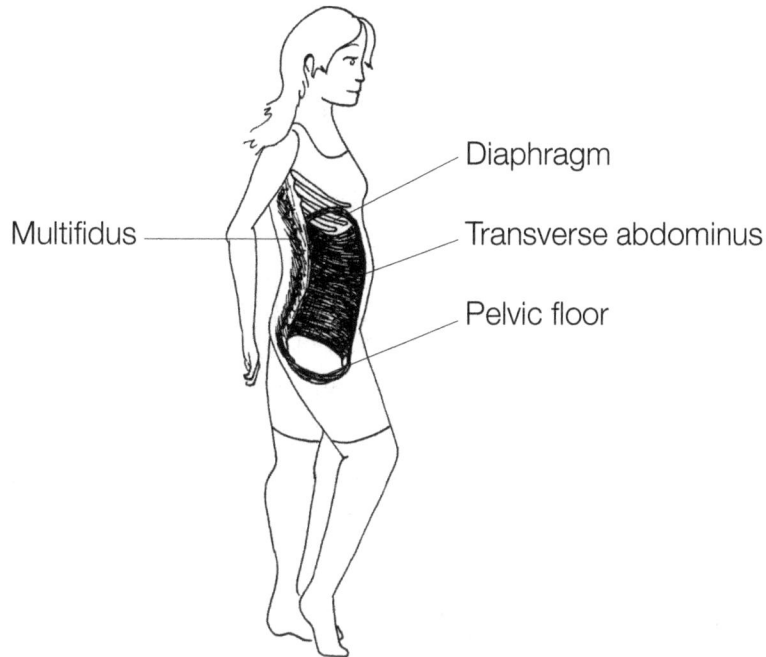

Figure 15. The core muscles

The top part of the inner core is the diaphragm. The pelvic floor muscles are at the bottom. Every time you breathe in, the pelvic floor muscles move down slightly; as you exhale they move up. The corset muscle is the transverse abdominus; as you breathe, it gently lengthens and shortens, moving slightly. As you begin to move, all of these muscles automatically activate.

The pelvic floor muscles arise from the tailbone (coccyx) and run all the way to the front, to the pubic bone. A simple way to think of these muscles is as a hammock which is secure at the back but has a little more give or stretch in the middle and at the front. Some of the pelvic muscles extend to each side and attach to the hip bones. Weak pelvic floor muscles can cause hip pain, and vice-versa. Further, a hip problem can prevent the pelvic floor muscles from engaging effectively, which can cause back pain.

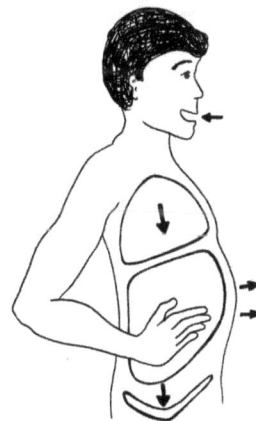

The pelvic floor muscles have fascial attachments to the transverse abdominus, the deepest abdominal muscle, which is under the external and internal oblique and rectus abdominus, often referred to as the six-pack.

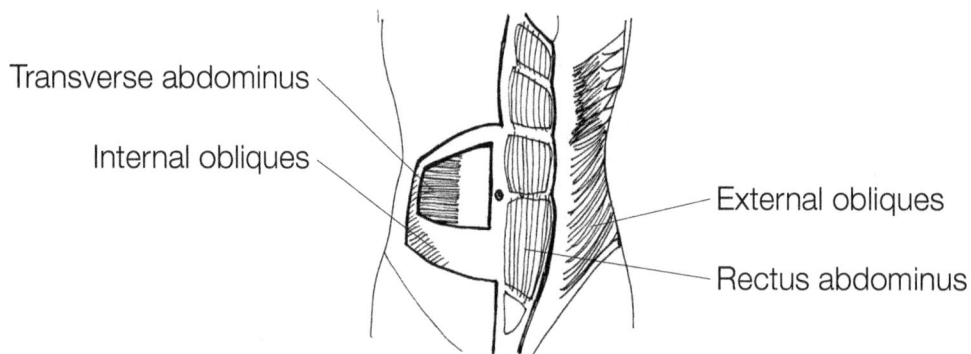

Figure 16. The transverse abdominus lies underneath the internal and external obliques and the rectus abdominus

The transverse abdominus wraps around the abdomen and joins at the back onto the deep segmental spinal muscles, the multifidus. The transverse abdominus encases the body as if a corset were placed around the waistline, with looser connections in the midline at the front.

This inner corset muscle has fascial attachments to the ribs and hip bones. Therefore stiffness in the mid back or hips could restrict the automatic engagement of the core muscles.

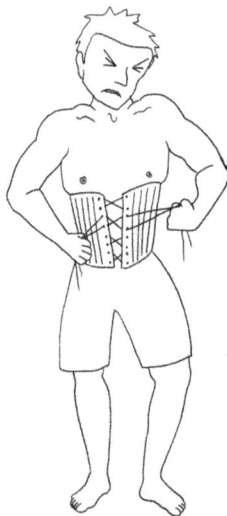

Feel your core muscles

If sitting, move as if you are about to stand up, but remain seated. You will feel your inner corset core muscles activate. You do not have to think about holding your abdominal organs in or stabilising your spine and other joints; that all takes place automatically.

When you have back pain, this automated action is delayed and that is why your back might lock at unpredictable times. The superficial power muscles are activating too quickly to compensate for weakness of the core muscles.

Knowing this is the essence of training the core. Learning how to do core exercises correctly, and getting these muscles to become engaged automatically again, is potentially one of the most important aspects you need to know to overcome your back pain.

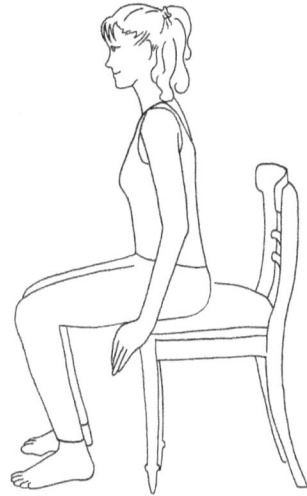

Real Time Ultrasound

If you have the opportunity I highly recommend you consult a health professional who uses Real Time Ultrasound imaging. This technology shows your inner muscles and enables the practitioner to identify and assess any weakness in your core muscles. This information will help you to learn how to do the core exercises correctly.

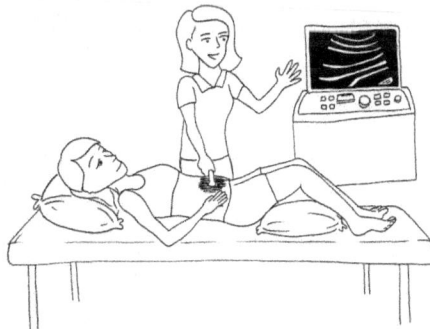

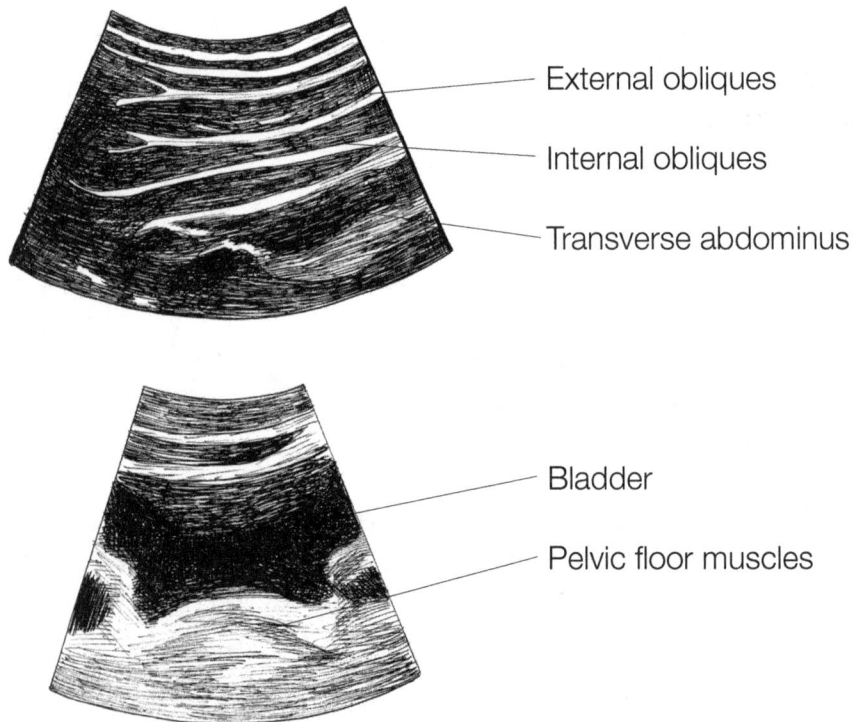

— External obliques

— Internal obliques

— Transverse abdominus

— Bladder

— Pelvic floor muscles

Figure 17. A Real Time Ultrasound (RTU) image shows the superficial external obliques and transverse abdominus. It also shows how the pelvic floor muscles look when scanned through the lower abdominals. Doing an RTU assessment with a physiotherapist is an excellent way to understand how the body works and to learn how to use transverse abdominus and pelvic floor muscles correctly

What the brain can tell us

The transverse abdominus registers in a different part of the brain when back pain is present.

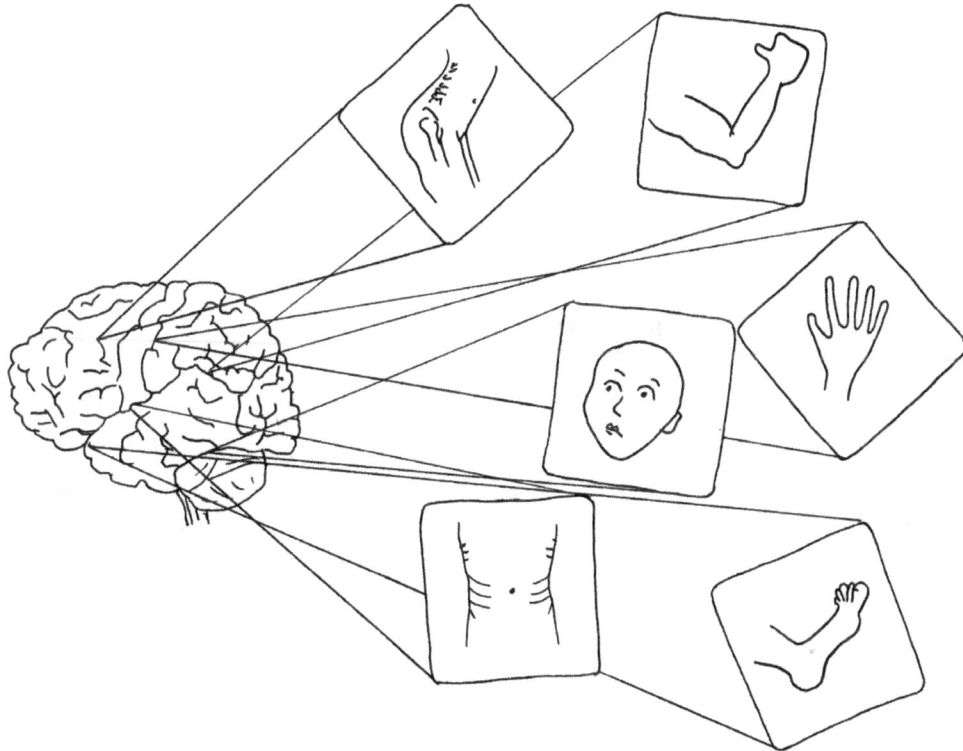

Figure 18. The homunculus is the area of the brain in which every structure of the body is represented or depicted. Research has shown that the representation of the transverse abdominus moves to a different part of the homunculus when back pain occurs. This finding supports what RTU imaging shows in the clinic. Exciting new research reveals that the changes in the brain can be reversed with specific transverse abdominus retraining. Such training would mean that this muscle would activate in the correct, automated way, as it did before you had back pain

SIX STEPS TO FIND AND ACTIVATE CORE MUSCLES

Step 1. Observe the abdominal muscles as you breathe

▶ Stand facing a mirror and watch your abdomen.

▶ Watch yourself breathing in and out. Notice that your abdomen extends outward as you breathe in and draws inward as you breathe out.

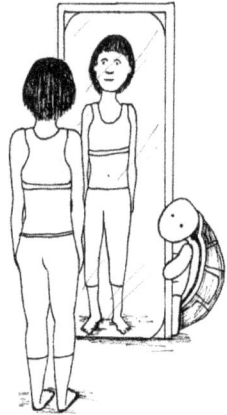

Step 2. Relax the neck and shoulders

▶ Check whether you can keep your neck and shoulders relaxed as you breathe, or if they rise upward. If you cannot keep your neck and shoulders relaxed, you could be breathing more into your upper airways. This can prevent your inner core muscles from working effectively.

▶ Soften your neck and shoulder muscles, relax them downward. Keep them in this relaxed position as you keep breathing lower into the abdomen.

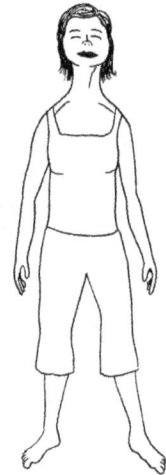

Step 3. Breathe into the diaphragm

Place your hands at the sides of your body on your lower rib cage. Feel the air fill up the space under each hand. Keep the neck and shoulders calm and relaxed. Imagine the air that you are taking in is broadening your back and lengthening your spine. This is called diaphragm breathing.

If you notice that your back has tightened after some activity, diaphragm breathing will often help loosen the tight muscles.

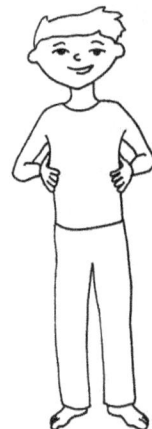

Step 4. Identify your upper and lower abdominals

▶ Can you see any difference between the abdominal muscles that are above the belly button and below it (the upper and lower abdominals)?

▶ You might see a hollow and tightness in your upper abdominals and they might look strong. However, you might be carrying a little extra weight and have less tone and strength in the muscles between the belly button and the pubic bone. If so, this usually shows that your inner core is weak.

▶ The remedy is to engage the lower abdominal muscles while relaxing and taking some of the tautness from the upper abdominals, as outlined below.

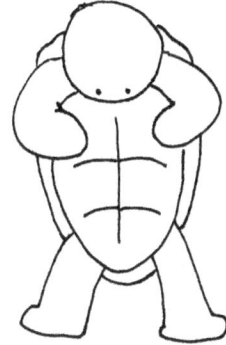

Here is how to engage the lower abdominals while relaxing the upper ones. Stand facing the mirror; keep your hands on your upper abdominals and try to keep those muscles relaxed. There is usually a small hollow just under your rib cage when you tense your upper abdominals. This is a good position to place your hands or the tips of your fingers.

Imagine that someone has tapped you gently on your chest and you fell backward a little. You will feel all of your abdominal muscles tighten. This will give you a sense of how your core muscles are automated and engaged with even the slightest movement.

When you repeat this movement, focus on engaging the lower abdominals while trying to keep the upper abdominals more relaxed.

Step 5. Engage the pelvic floor muscles

▶ Keep the upper abdominals relaxed and engage your pelvic floor muscles. You should feel activation of your lower abdominals.

▶ If you are unsure how to engage your pelvic floor muscles, imagine you were stopping yourself mid-stream when urinating. This will give you a sense of where your pelvic floor muscles are.

▶ Imagine that you are getting into a lift and keep your pelvic floor muscles engaged as though you were only going to the first level. Do not over-tense the muscles or do a maximum contraction. Try to do five breaths with neck and shoulders relaxed while the pelvic floor muscles are still gently engaged.

▶ Women should use a squeezing action, which strengthens the sphincters of the pelvic floor, as well doing a lifting contraction.

▶ Men should lift the pelvic floor towards the belly button. This has been shown to be an effective cue to engage these muscles correctly.

The important thing is not to keep doing a maximum contraction of your pelvic floor muscles continually throughout the day. This could create other problems. The gentle contraction is the one that starts to activate the other core muscles correctly. This is called a sub-maximal contraction as opposed to a maximum contraction. It is certainly a good thing to do a maximum contraction, but only once a day. This is usually sufficient to look after the strength of the sphincters of the pelvic floor.

Note: If you have specific pelvic floor issues or you are unsure how to do pelvic floor exercises, please do consult a physiotherapist who specialises in this particular area of health.

Step 6. Exercise the feet and thighs

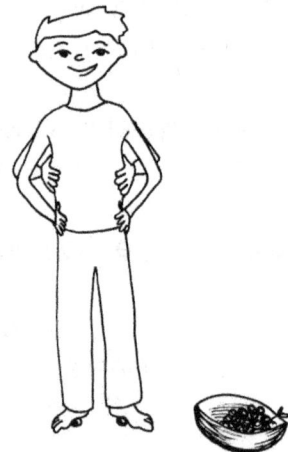

▶ Imagine that there is a grape under the arch of each foot. With a very small movement, lift your arches up and off the grape, and turn the feet slightly outward.

▶ Also imagine wrapping the thighs outward around the thigh bone.

▶ Be sure to keep the first (big) toe on the ground and do not clench all your other toes.

▶ Soften the neck and shoulders and keep them relaxed.

Observe whether doing these small movements with your feet and thighs has any effect on your posture or your core muscles. If you see that it does, doing these small awareness movements during the day will help correct your posture. If it feels too tiring to lift your arches, this might show a need to wear shoes with more arch support. You might need custom-made orthotics to support your back and posture a little more.

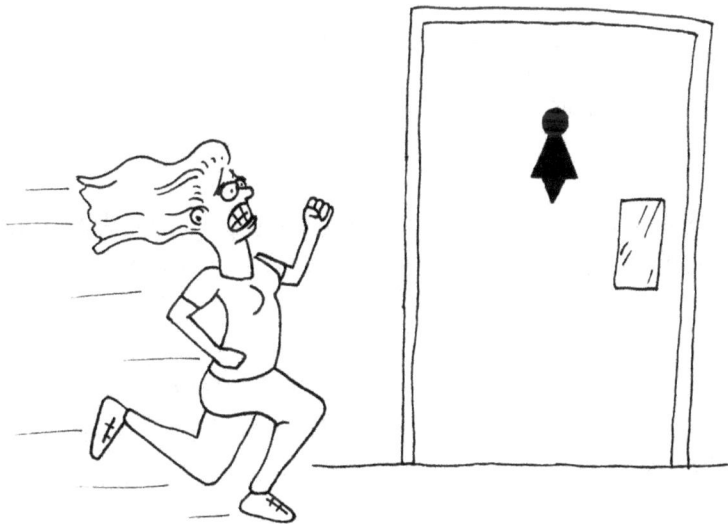

"I wondered why I have to race and pee sometimes – maybe it's my weak pelvic floor muscles?"

How to identify weak pelvic floor muscles

You could have weak pelvic floor muscles if you:

▶ experience episodes of leaking or stress incontinence when you sneeze or cough

▶ have urge incontinence; that is, you need to go to the toilet urgently and the urge is hard to control

▶ have had gynaecological, urological or abdominal surgery

▶ are overweight

▶ experience cardio-respiratory problems (for instance asthma) that overwork the upper respiratory muscles around the neck and shoulders and can therefore compromise the pelvic floor muscles, or

▶ have had a baby, recently or many years ago. If you have had more than three children, there is a high correlation between back pain and weakened pelvic floor muscles.

If you are unsure of how to contract your pelvic floor muscles, you should consult a physiotherapist who can assess these muscles with RTU imaging through the abdomen.

Some women might need an internal assessment to be sure of engaging these muscles correctly. A physiotherapist who specialises in women's health is the appropriate person to consult for this check.

There are references in the recommended reading if you want to understand and read more on this highly important topic.

Strengthening pelvic floor muscles is often one of the most important factors in resolving longstanding back or hip pain.

Wake up your core muscles while walking

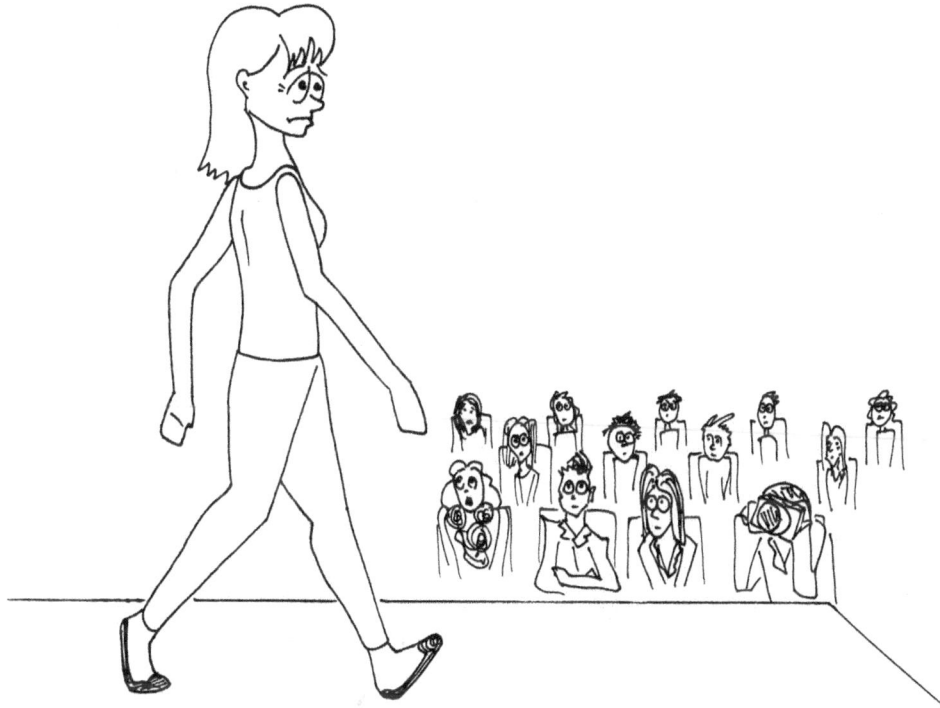

"Why is everyone looking at me?"

When you are in pain it is so easy to slump. But this perpetuates poor muscle habits and prolongs your back pain. When you walk along the street, see how many people are looking at the ground, at their phone or at their feet. Use the simple tips you learned for engaging your core when standing; put them into action while walking. Think tall but stay relaxed; even this small movement will help automate your core. People will notice your improved posture.

Home exercise: balancing the books

This exercise is one of the best ways to connect with your stability muscles and improve your posture.

Place a book on top of your head and walk in a straight line. Make the exercise more challenging by placing one foot directly in front of the other. This is often called the sobriety test. You will be surprised how hard it is. Difficulty in balancing and stabilising your weight over each foot shows that you need to strengthen your core muscles.

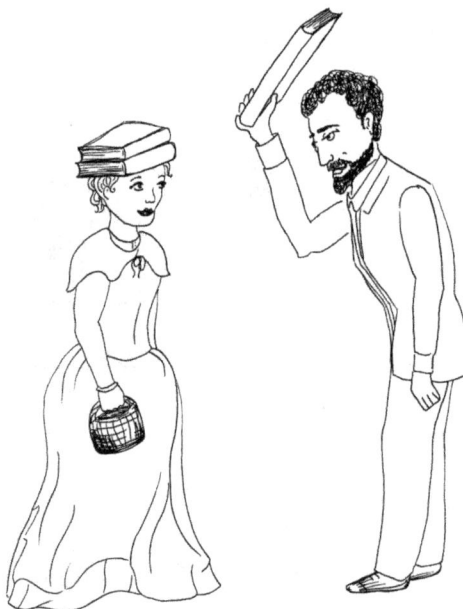

Poor balance can often come from weak postural and stability muscles. Take care to do this exercise close to a wall if you know that your balance is not good.

How "flutter" can activate your stability muscles

Research has shown that if you move your arm or your hand while engaging your stability muscles it encourages these muscles to stay engaged. This provides endurance training for these muscles, which helps prevent postural fatigue. This peripheral limb movement is called "perturbation". For simplicity I call it "flutter".

Shake your hand repetitively, as if shaking water off your fingers, while your core is engaged. Keep your elbow straight. Do not brace your abdominals. Shake one hand at a time. You can easily do this exercise while sitting or standing. The exercise cannot be done in a slumped posture, which is why it is so beneficial. While in a lazy posture, the hand will not be able to do this repetitive movement.

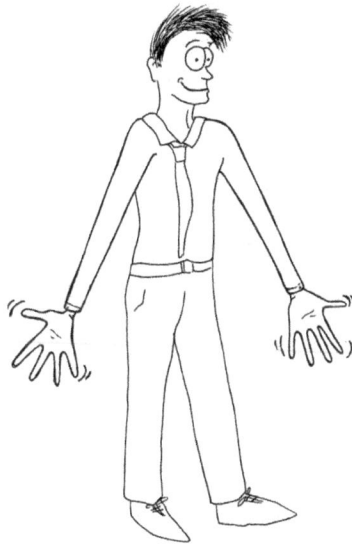

"I think this flutter movement is great! I have to stand taller
and adopt a better posture to keep this movement going"

To understand why this hand movement assists the core, think about picking up a cup of tea. You do not have to think about keeping your shoulder in its socket, where your mouth is and so on; all these actions are automated. That is what we are trying to achieve by fluttering. Your stability muscles activate to enable the hand movement, otherwise your whole body would wobble.

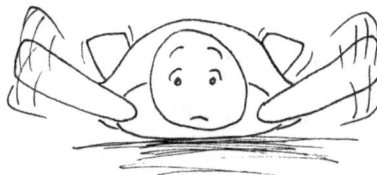

"Can't say this flutter thing is working for me..."

Postural sway to activate your core

Doing a small swaying movement can activate your core muscles. It should not be discernible to anybody next to you. Relax the upper abdominals as you do this small swaying movement. Place your fingers in the hollow on either side of the midline under the rib cage to monitor this. Next place your hands behind into the small of the back. Try to relax the superficial strong muscles, the erector spinae; this will encourage the deeper stability muscles to engage.

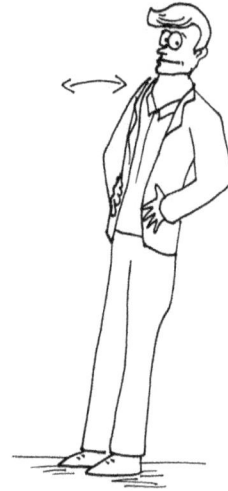

"I'm waking up my core muscles
- I hope nobody notices"

Waking up core muscles while you sit

The cues that apply to standing and walking to activate your core also apply to sitting. Try adding in these steps:

▸ Find the centre of gravity over your sitting bones. Visualise separating your sitting bones and then drawing them together. This will alert you to where your pelvic floor muscles are when you are sitting.

▸ Think tall, but be sure to relax the neck and shoulders and deliberately breathe into the diaphragm.

▸ Arch and flatten the back and then bring your spine into a position that feels centred. This is often called spinal neutral.

▸ Imagine that you are about to stand; initiate the movement ever so slightly. You will feel your core muscles activate. Consciously keep them engaged for five breaths. You will benefit from repeating this exercise every hour or so to prevent postural fatigue if you have a sedentary job. Remember it is only a very minimal movement. The only thing a person sitting next to you should notice is that you have excellent posture and are not slumped.

▸   Remember to flutter each hand in turn.

Good posture is not about being rigid, but about everything being calm, relaxed and balanced. With regular prompts and by correcting your posture, you will be able to maintain good posture for much longer without tiring or needing to slump.

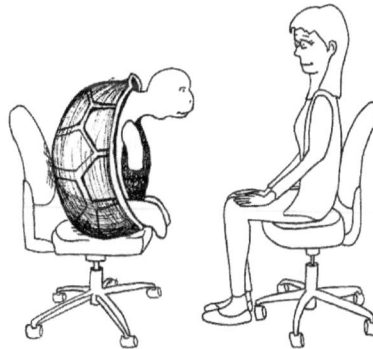

"I think she's doing this better than me"

Singing can help reduce pain

If you are still unsure about where your core muscles are, try this: while sitting, place your hands on your abdomen and start humming. You will feel your abdominal muscles engage. But do not keep humming. Hum a little; stop humming and relax; then hum again. Singing can help reduce pain, so are you game to do this in public? Perhaps you should be selective about when you do some singing or the humming exercise.

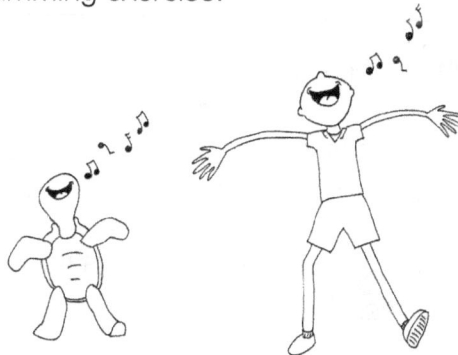

Mistakes to avoid with core stability

▶ Do not brace or merely suck in your stomach

▶ Do not tense your neck and shoulders

▶ Do not use only the upper abdominals

▶ Do not flatten your back too much

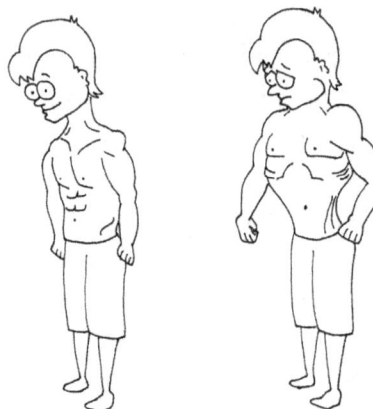

Here are the four common mistakes to avoid when doing core stability exercises.

Bracing the stomach: Doing core exercises does not mean sucking in all of your abdominal muscles at once. Some of my patients do this when they are trying to look thinner, but this practice stiffens the superficial back muscles and can cause more back pain.

Tensing neck and shoulders: Watch the strap muscle at the front of your neck and your upper shoulder muscles as you face a mirror and engage your core muscles. These should all be relaxed as you do core exercises, whether you stand, sit or lie down. Be careful not to hold your breath. Keep breathing deeply into your lungs to expand your diaphragm. This will also help you relax your neck and shoulders.

Over-using the upper abdominals: Watch your reflection and observe whether the upper abdominals tighten and tense up first when you engage your inner core. The correct technique is to engage the lower abdominals, which "corset" the lower back, before engaging the upper abdominals.

Flattening the back: When lying down during stability exercises, do not flatten your back too much. Keep the back in soft contact with the floor as you do core exercises. Arch your back and then flatten it to find a position half-way between the two extremes. Choose the position at which your back feels most supported and comfortable. In the correct position you should feel no pain.

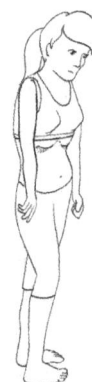

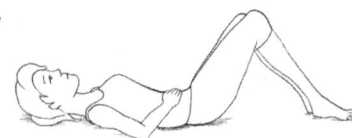

Use a mirror to observe your core muscles

If you are still unsure about whether you are engaging your core correctly, doing this exercise on your hands and knees will enable you to feel and observe the core muscles working. Start with totally relaxing all of your abdominals. Do not protrude the stomach downward or excessively arch the back up. Keep your spine straight, as in the illustration below. Think about and initiate a move to lift your hand off the floor. You will easily feel your abdominals engage. Do this with your other hand, relax it again, and initiate slightly lifting each knee. Concentrate on breathing comfortably as you lift each hand or knee.

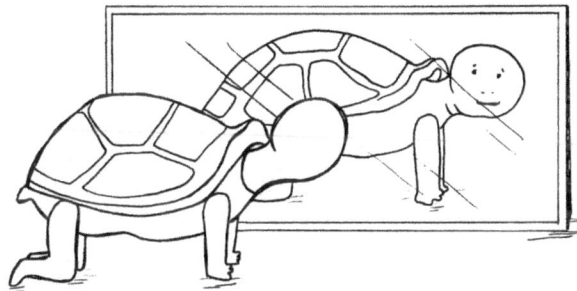

Try these movements sidelong to a mirror. You can easily check whether your lower abdominals are engaging before your upper abdominals. That is the correct sequence for engaging your core muscles. First, let all of your abdominal muscles relax; breathe in, and as you exhale, focus on engaging your pelvic floor and lower abdominals. Do not hold your breath; keep your spine straight. Take five relaxed breaths while the lower abdominals are engaged, without tightening up anywhere else in your body. Keep your neck and shoulders relaxed, even though you will find this challenging.

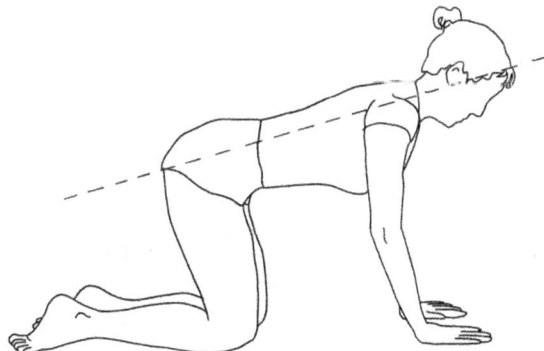

Lessons learned from astronauts

We have learned a lot from astronauts about how to manage and treat back pain. When in space, they develop muscle weakness among many health problems. In the back and other joints in the body, astronauts' muscles atrophied or weakened in a specific order. This was also associated with poor core stability and poor balance. These findings are the same as the muscle weakness that is associated with back pain. Retraining the inner core and stability muscles is an integral component to improving astronauts' balance and strength when they are no longer in an antigravity environment. Much of this stability and strength training correlates with our current management and treatment of back pain.

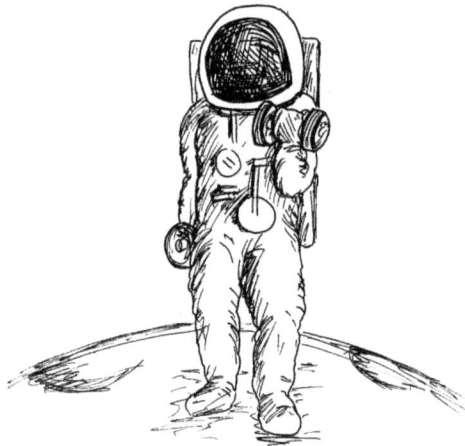

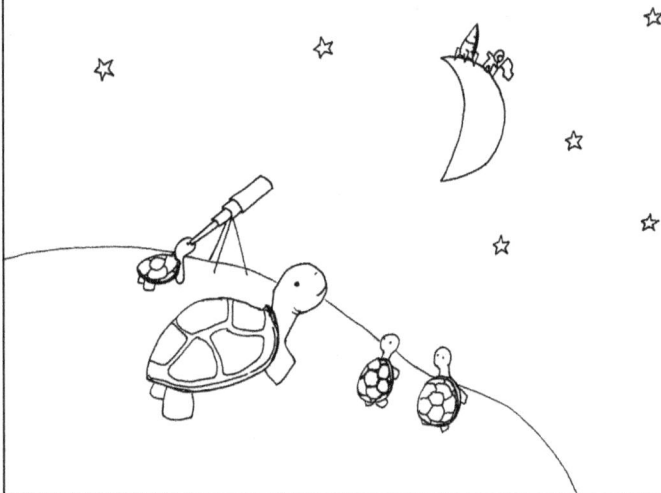

"Isn't that amazing kids? We've learned how to help back pain from the man on the moon"

CORE STABILITY SELF-TESTS

Now that you have located your core muscles, it is time to start training them to do a better job.

Begin with two tests to check whether you have an imbalance between the core muscles on either side of your body. This will enable you to focus on your weaker side during the exercises. With back pain it is quite normal to have a difference in strength between the sides of your body. Your daily habits in standing, sitting and other postures contribute to any imbalance.

Two key tests are the standing heel raise and the gentle leg lift or active straight leg raise. Do two to three repetitions only, on each side.

⚠ **CAUTION:** If you are experiencing an acute episode of back pain, let your back settle before you do these tests. Likewise if you feel pain while doing either test, cease it immediately.

Test 1. Standing on one leg and raising the heel

Place your second and third finger only onto a desk or a table for balance. Stand on one leg with the other one raised off the floor. Do you need to clench your toes or drop into one side more than the other? If you are unsure, close your eyes and check whether it is harder to keep your balance on one side than the other. Note which is your weaker side.

Raising heels to test stability: Raise the heel of each foot independently. Do not use your arms to help you. Maintain only finger contact with the table. Repeat this two or three times on each side. The side on which the test is more difficult to do and requires more lateral movement or wobbling, is likely to be your weaker side.

Your pain might not be on your weaker side; this is not uncommon. Usually this means that the pain you are experiencing is caused by tight muscles compensating for your weaker side.

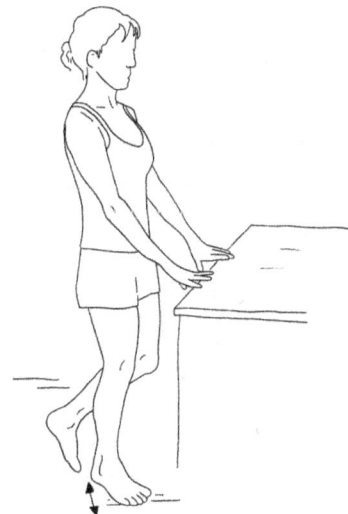

If you are still uncertain whether the two sides of your body feel different, try the second test.

Test 2. Gentle leg lift

Lying on your back, place your hands on your hips and feel the hip bone. Now rest your fingers on the muscle beside this bone. Think about lifting one leg off the floor; initiate the movement for a few centimetres only. One leg might feel heavier than the other and the pelvis will drop on that side; this is the weaker side. When you do your stability exercises, be aware of this drop. Try to engage the core a little more on that side to correct the drop, but do not brace the muscles.

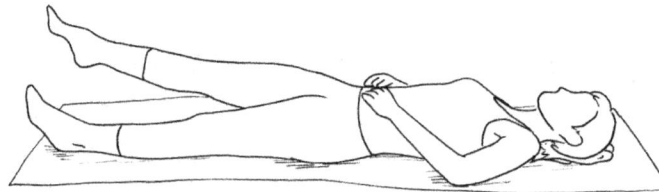

You might notice improvement in your leg lift after about 10 days of stability exercises, providing you do not revert to imbalanced postural habits.

Do the second test every 10 days, but not more often. Remember: It is not an exercise; it is a test.

Gentle leg lift to test stability

Helpful tip: Always start core exercises on your stronger side first, then move to the weaker side.

Starting core exercises on your stronger side trains the brain on how to do the exercise. Do twice as many repetitions on the weaker side. To finish off a routine, do one exercise each on the left and right and focus on whether they are starting to feel more even. Do the first test each week to gauge whether your balance and stability are improving.

Points to remember

▶ Core muscles refer to the diaphragm, pelvic floor muscles, transverse abdominus and multifidus.

▶ These are the muscles that pre-activate when you are about to move; they stabilise your back and support the abdominal organs.

▶ One or all of these muscles can be compromised or weakened after even one episode of back pain.

▶ Core exercises done incorrectly can cause back pain instead of alleviating it.

▶ Using your hand with a fluttering movement can stimulate the core muscles; fluttering during the day can prevent postural fatigue.

▶ Doing a small postural sway movement can help your core muscles to activate.

▶ You need to relax your back muscles and breathe freely when doing fluttering or postural sway exercises.

Actions to take

Standing in front of a mirror, take these six steps to identify and engage the core muscles correctly:

▶ Observe your breathing.

▶ Relax neck and shoulders.

▶ Practice diaphragm breathing.

▶ Relax your upper abdominals and engage the lower abdominals.

▶ Engage your pelvic floor muscles and observe how this affects the lower abdominal muscles.

▶ Lift the arches of your feet and initiate the movement of turning your feet outwards. As you do this, imagine you are wrapping your thigh muscle outwards and around the thigh bone (femur).

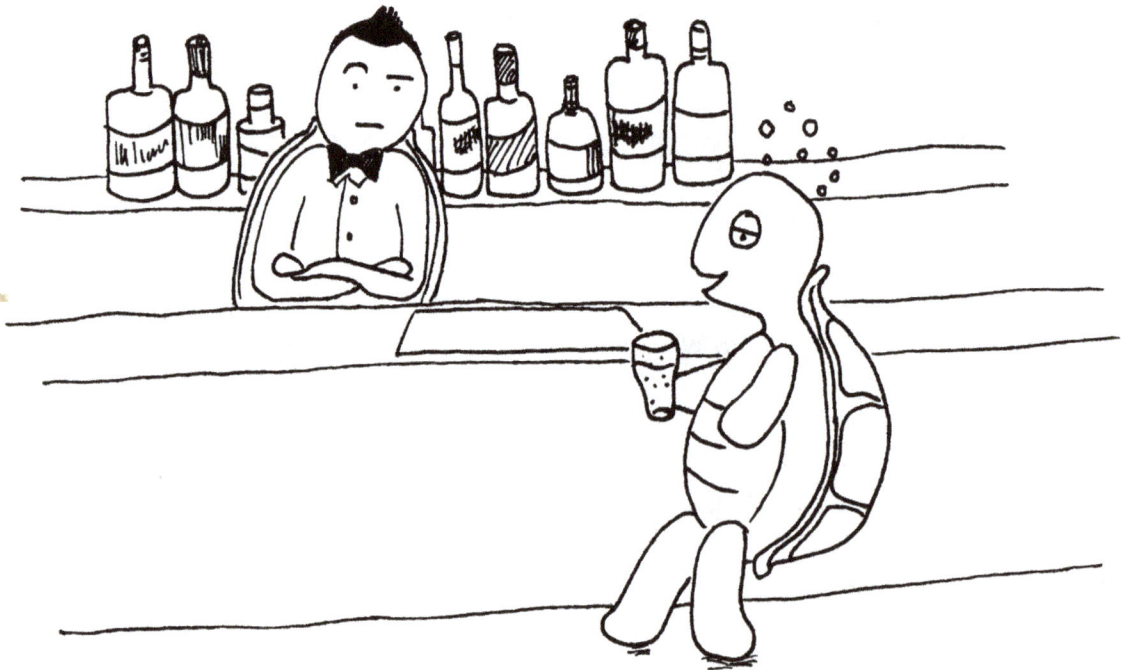

"This swaying thing is really easy...I wonder if my core is working... maybe not..."

Notes

6 Core stability exercises

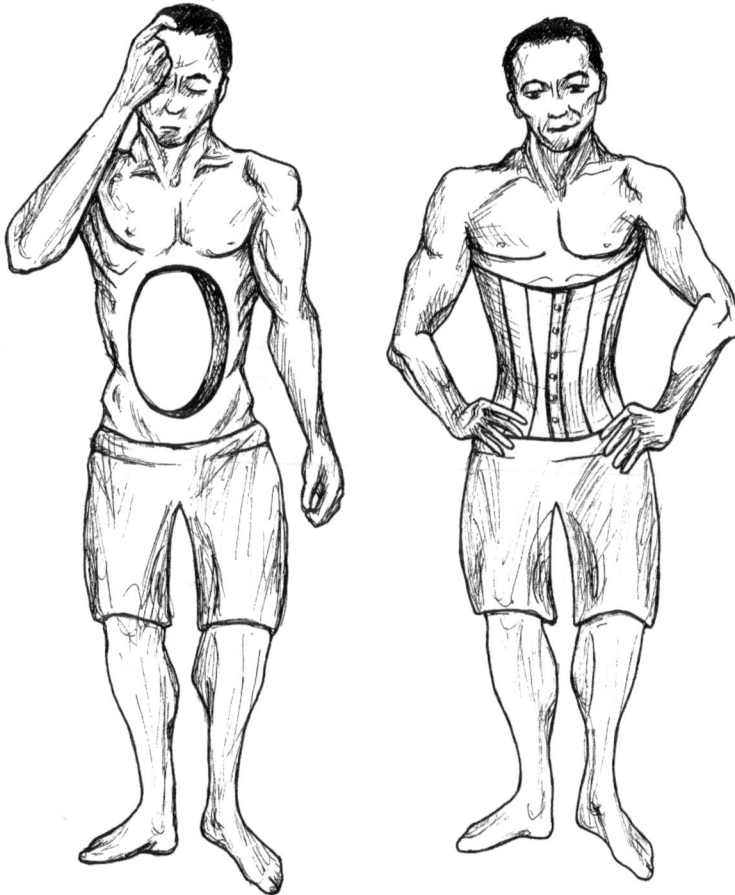

"Can't I just have a corset instead of doing these exercises for muscles I can't even see?"

Now you have learned where the core muscles are and how to engage them correctly, you are ready to start doing core exercises. You can start gently with breathing, keeping the neck and shoulders relaxed, then engage the pelvic floor muscles and transverse abdominus. At first, these exercises are best done while lying down; you can then progress to doing them while standing or on hands and knees.

When you begin these exercises you might need to stop and practise each one. The goal, however, is to have each exercise flowing from one to the next. Level one should eventually only take you about 10 to 15 minutes. If you finish them more quickly than this you are not doing them correctly. Remember the overall goal is to know the location of your core muscles. With pain they have become inhibited. After a while you should not need to think about the core muscles all the time; they will automatically respond and activate each time you go to move. Nevertheless, you need to consciously engage your core if you are doing heavy or unpredictable lifting (for instance, your children).

LEVEL 1. CORE STABILITY EXERCISES

Exercise 9. Abdominal breathing

Lying on your back, place one hand on your chest and the other on your lower abdomen. Relax your neck, shoulders and jaw. Breathe in and notice whether your chest rises before your abdomen. Practise relaxing the chest and letting the abdomen rise and fall as you breathe in a relaxed manner. This is called abdominal breathing; it helps your brain to connect with your inner core muscles. Place your hands laterally on each side of your rib cage and try to breathe deeply into this area of your body. Repeat this exercise for two or three minutes.

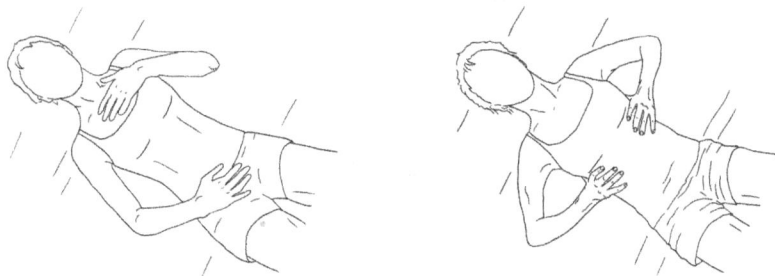

Exercise 10. Spinal neutral

While lying on your back, arch the back a little, then flatten. Find a position somewhere between arching and flattening that feels the most comfortable and relaxed. We call this spinal neutral. It is the best position in which to locate and retrain your stability muscles.

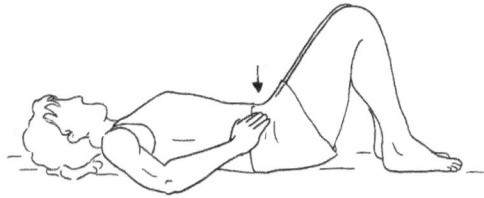

Exercise 11. Engaging the pelvic floor muscles

Place your hands just inside the front hip bone onto the lower abdominal muscles. If the pelvic floor muscles are engaged, you should feel a small amount of muscle tension under your fingers. Breathe in; as you breathe out, engage the pelvic floor muscles. It is helpful to think of a muscle running from your tailbone or coccyx through to your pubic bone at the front. So that you do not overdo this contraction, think of being in a lift and taking the pelvic floor muscles up to level one, still breathing; then level two, and up to level four or five. The goal is to keep the pelvic floor muscles engaged at each level and to continue breathing comfortably, not tensing the neck and shoulders and not holding your breath. Try this challenge: hold the pelvic floor muscle engaged for five to ten breaths (at each level).

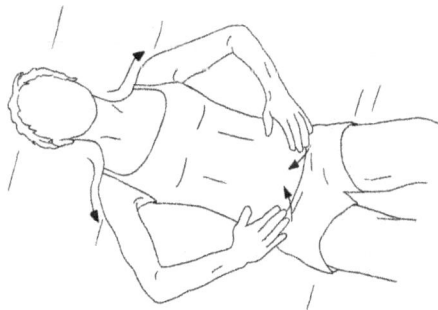

Exercise 12. Pelvic floor muscles plus transverse abdominus

Lying on your back with your knees bent and your feet on the ground, continue abdominal breathing. Place your hands on your hips with your fingertips right next to the hip bone (the ilium). Breathe in; as you breathe out engage your pelvic floor muscles, focusing on your lower abdomen. You should feel your lower abdominals engage. Maintain this contraction while you do five to ten diaphragm breaths. To test whether you are doing this correctly, initiate lifting your hips off the ground as you exhale. You will feel maximum engagement of your abdominals as you do this. Lower the intensity of this movement until you are only using five per cent of the effort you needed to do this. The goal is to maintain this low-level contraction for the duration of five to ten breaths.

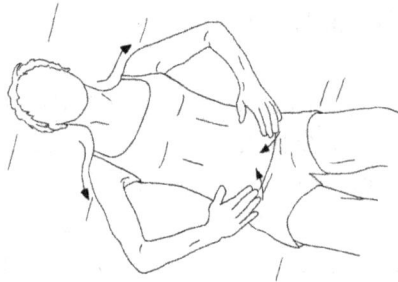

Exercise 13. Pelvic floor and transverse abdominus with leg drop-out

Lying on your back, maintain relaxed abdominal breathing. As you exhale, allow one knee to drop out to the side at an angle of about 20 to 30 degrees. If one leg feels wobbly as it drops to the side, imagine a few grains of sand slowly running from the top of your knee down deep into the ball and socket of the hip. This can assist in recruiting the deep hip stability muscles. You should not be hitching your hip. That is, an observer should not be able to see that you are engaging your deep hip muscles. Repeat four to five times on each leg.

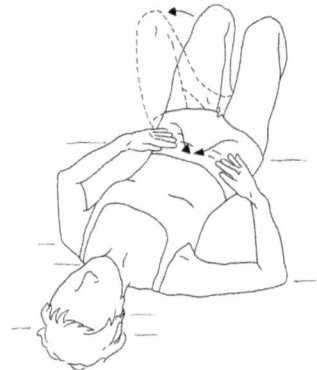

Exercise 14. Simultaneously contracting pelvic floor and transverse abdominus muscles

An excellent way of knowing whether you are engaging your lower abdominals before your upper abdominals is to go onto your hands and knees with your body sidelong to a mirror, the position you adopted when locating the core muscles. You can use it to engage the core muscles for a little longer. Watch in the mirror as you breathe in and out. You will see your abdomen move down as you breathe in and up as you breathe out. Now think of lifting a hand off the floor. Repeat this with your other hand and then each knee. You will feel the core activate as you are about to start this movement. Do not lift hand or knee off the floor; just initiate the smallest movement as though you were going to lift.

Next, engage your pelvic floor muscles. See whether this affects your lower abdominals. It should. If you notice that only your upper abdominals are contracting, relax them. As you engage the pelvic floor muscles, try to activate the lower abdominals before the upper abdominals. Take care not to hold your breath as the inner core is engaged. Maintain ideal back alignment, not curved up, flexed or extended down. Take five to ten breaths, while the pelvic floor and transverse abdominus muscles are engaged.

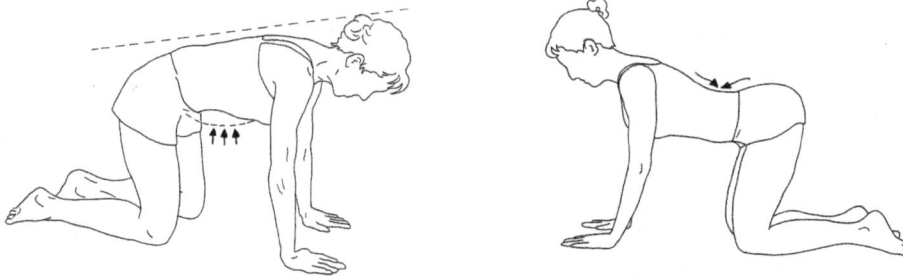

Stability exercises while standing

Once you think you have mastered engaging the core muscles while lying down, the next step is to practise engaging them while standing. It is important to link doing the deep inner core abdominal muscles and feel how these connect with the stability muscles in the back.

Exercise 15. Postural sway, locating the multifidus muscle

Place your hands behind your back and rest the
pads of your fingers on the bony prominences in the
midline of your back. These are called the spinous
processes. Bend (flex) and arch your spine a little
and this will help you find this part of your spine. Now
let your fingers move off the spinous processes into
the hollow next to the spine. This is where the deep
muscle multifidus is located. If you feel a really tight
strong muscle (erector spinae) under your fingers,
you have moved too far outwards away from the
spine. You may recall we called these the two rods of
muscle that go into protective spasm with back pain
or weakness of the core.

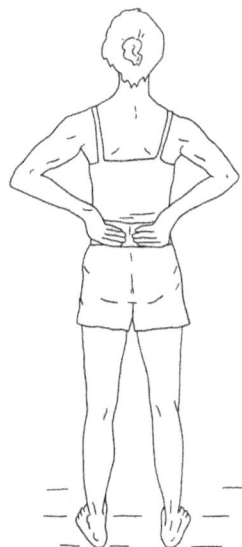

Keep your weight evenly distributed over each foot while you sway forward and
back a little, from heel to toe. It is a very small movement and would be barely
visible to someone next to you. Multifidus will be working, even if you are not
sure that it is, provided you keep the strong superficial erector spinae muscles
as relaxed as possible and keep your spine upright and supported.

If you are still uncertain whether you are doing this exercise correctly, engage
your pelvic floor muscles and transverse abdominus while you keep the long
erector spinae muscles relaxed. All these muscles work together to provide the
support your spine needs when you go to move.

It is helpful to do postural sway in front of a mirror to be sure that you do not
brace your upper abdominals; they will show a distinct hollow if you do brace
them. This is wrong and will cause your superficial erector spinae muscles to
tighten up.

Maintaining your height and good posture, think tall, relax the neck and
shoulders and repeat this swaying movement four or five times; rest and repeat
the process two or three times.

This exercise is helpful if your back aches after you have been standing for a long
time, or when you need to sit for an extended period.

Exercise 16. Multifidus with flutter and arm raise

The goal of this exercise is to keep the core muscles including multifidus engaged as you do a repetitive flutter movement with one hand. This is called perturbation. The repetitive movement prompts the core muscles to engage. If they are not engaged, your whole body will wobble as you do this movement. Keep the flutter movement going for 20 to 30 seconds. Do it with each hand independently and monitor the muscles on the opposite side of your back.

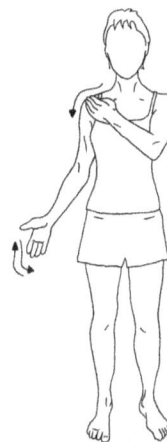

If you cannot feel the deep back muscles or are unsure whether they are working, keep one hand on the superficial erector spinae muscles of the back while you raise the other hand. If you feel these superficial muscles tighten up the moment you raise your arm, you are doing the exercise correctly. The goal is to keep the erector spinae muscles as relaxed as possible while you repeat either the flutter movement or the arm raise movement. Keep the thumb facing upwards at about 45 degrees away from the body when doing the arm raise, and repeat four or five times on each side.

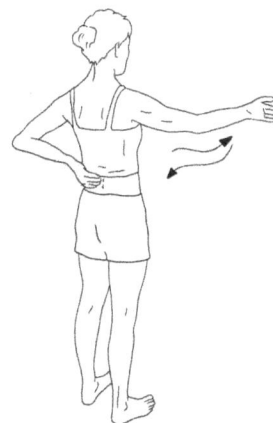

LEVEL 2. INTERMEDIATE STABILITY EXERCISES

If you can now competently do all the Level 1 exercises, it is time to progress. The goal now is to train the core muscles to stay engaged as you move either your arms or legs. This makes the core exercises more challenging.

Supine stability using the arms and legs

Exercise 17. Leg slide

While lying on your back, knees bent, engage the pelvic floor and transverse abdominus and slide the leg outwards and then back to the start position.

Maintain spinal neutral; that is, do not excessively flatten your back. Keep the core muscles gently engaged. Do not let the leg collapse outwards onto the ground. It is best to start with simply initiating the movement, extending the leg away from the body by only eight to ten centimetres. Once you can achieve this easily with the core still engaged, progress to extending the leg fully. Alternate each leg. Repeat four to five times on each side.

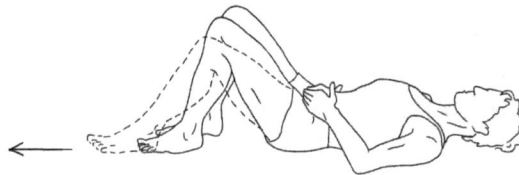

Exercise 18. Leg slides with arms raised

Progression: Raise the arms at right-angles to the body and continue to extend one leg and then the other.

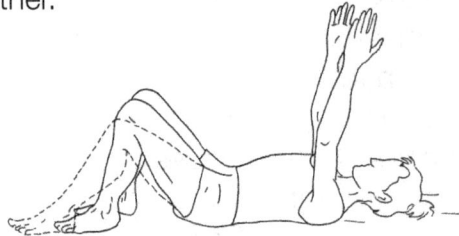

Exercise 19. Leg float

Return your hands to your lower abdomen; breathe in; as you exhale, float one leg up with knee bent, and return to the start position. Try not to press through the opposite foot as you do this; maintain an even pelvis, which means trying not to tilt and drop to one side; keep the core gently engaged throughout the exercise. Imagine that you have a cup of water on your abdomen and you do not want it to spill; this can help you not to let your pelvis tilt to either side.

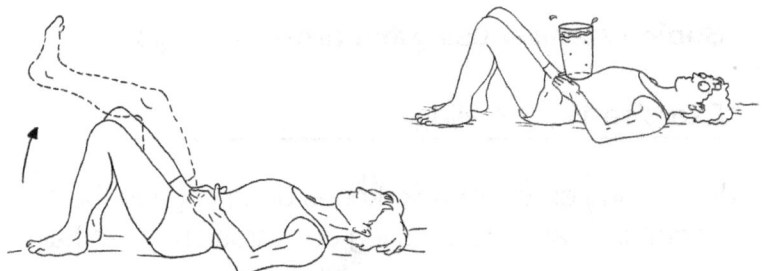

Exercise 20. Leg float with arms

Extend your arms at right-angles to the floor. Be sure to draw your shoulders back and down to engage the muscles between the shoulder-blades. Engage your core muscles and then float one leg off the ground and place it back down again. Repeat this on the opposite leg; keep repeating, three to six times with each leg. Exhale as you float the leg; try to use your hip flexors, the muscles at the front of your thigh, as little as possible. Put minimal pressure on the foot that remains on the ground.

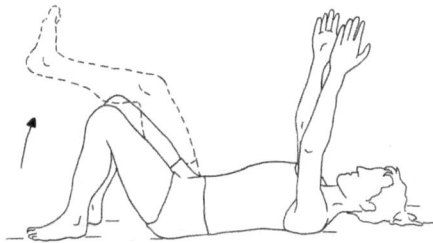

Exercise 21. Opposite arm and leg

Raise the arms at right-angles to the body. Float one leg off the ground and bring the shin bone parallel to the ground. Gently lift the other leg so that both legs and both arms are off the ground, still with your core muscles engaged. Be careful not to let your back arch as you extend your arm above your head; slowly lower the opposite leg, stopping just short of the floor. Repeat six to eight times on each side.

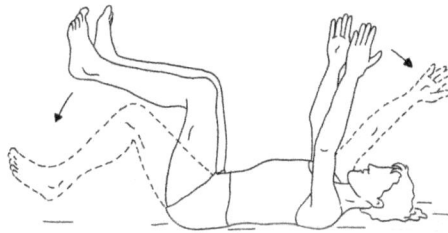

Prone stability exercises

Doing exercises while lying prone is an excellent way to find any muscle imbalance on either side of your body. If you have pain on one side of your body, you will find it harder to keep the gluteal muscles activated on that side. You might need to place your hands on your gluteal muscles to detect any imbalance. If you notice that one side is a lot weaker and you cannot feel this muscle working, repeat the exercise twice on the weaker side for every repetition you do on the stronger side. Relax your neck and shoulder muscles as you do all of the following exercises.

Exercise 22. Prone stability with knee bend

While lying prone, rest your forehead on the back of your hands; keep your neck and shoulders relaxed. Breathe in; as you exhale, bend one knee, then return it to a relaxed position. Repeat four or five times on each side. You might find that your hip hitches up as you do the exercise on one side; that is, the movement is not smooth. This usually shows that the hip flexor on that side is tight. Try a hip flexor stretch (see Chapter 7) and then return to this exercise. You should find it easier to do. When you bend one knee, the gluteal on that side should engage. However, do not tense the muscle too much; gently engage it as you bend your knee.

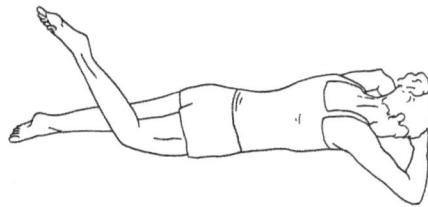

Eventually you want both sides to feel even, as you bend your knee.

Progression: If it feels too easy simply bending the knee, progress to bending the knee then lifting the leg a few millimetres off the ground and placing it down. You should not feel pain in your back when you do this exercise. The goal is to get both sides of your body to work more evenly. If you have had back pain or postural habits such as standing with all your weight on one leg, the sides of your body will usually be uneven. Repeat five times on each side. If you detect a weaker side, do two repetitions on your strong side and five on the weaker side.

Exercise 23: Engaging multifidus while focusing on diaphragm breathing

This exercise is a bit more challenging and you usually need a physiotherapist to check that you are doing it correctly. But give it a try.

Lie face down and place your hands around and onto your lower back. Locate the spinous processes and then put your fingers between this bony prominence and the superficial back extensors, the erector spinae, as you did for Exercise 16. Arch and flatten your back, then find a position in which the erector spinae are relaxed. Now breathe in and out, and as you exhale, engage your pelvic floor and transverse abdominus muscles and see whether you can feel a small contraction under your fingers. It is a subtle sensation of the muscle thickening under your fingers. The goal is to engage the multifidus muscle before the erector spinae contracts, and then maintain this contraction while you keep breathing laterally into your diaphragm four or five times.

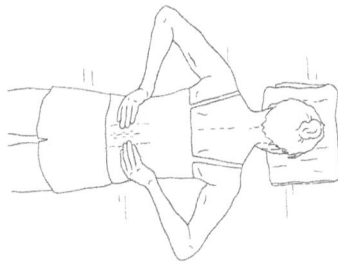

If you are not sure whether the multifidus muscle is working, try shortening or lengthening your leg. Either of these actions can activate the multifidus. Do not hitch the hip excessively; just do a very small movement. This can often help you locate the deep back-stabilising muscle, the multifidus.

Exercise 24. Four-point kneel with opposite arm and leg

Go down onto your hands and knees and maintain the natural curves of your spine; that is, do not arch too far up or down. Breathe in; as you exhale, engage your deep core muscles. First, think of lifting one knee a few millimetres off the ground but do not lift it. Think of lifting the opposite hand, but do not lift it. You will feel your deep core muscles engage. Progress this static exercise by engaging the core as you slide one leg out behind you, then raise it off the ground. Extend the opposite arm out to the side. Maintain this position on each side for five breaths.

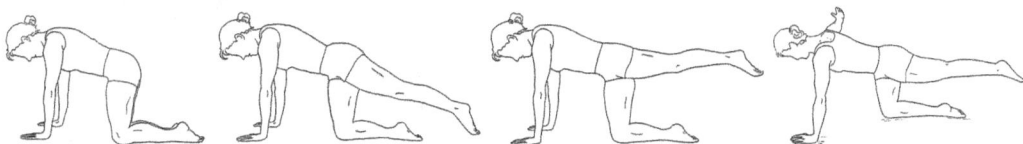

 Notes from the clinic

"I do competitive sport. Are the core exercises you have recommended too basic for me?"

Most sports injuries to muscle, tendon and bone are, aside from contact sports, due to overtraining, inappropriate equipment or poor biomechanics. Research shows that most hip, knee, foot and shoulder pain caused by playing sport is due to weakness of the stability muscles that support these joints. Irrespective of your fitness level, the starting point is to improve your core stability muscles then to add exercises specific to your sport.

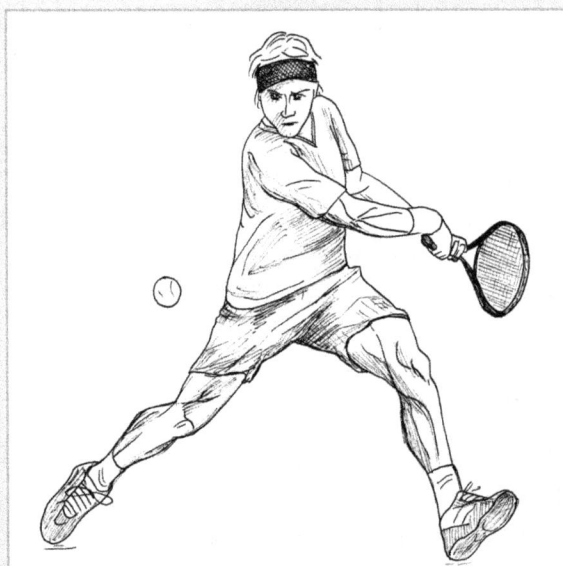

Do a quick postural assessment (Chapter 2) to assess how good you think your stability is, then identify your postural type (see Chapter 9). This is a great starting point for preventing or overcoming an injury. You will easily be able to design your own flexibility and strengthening program. However, if you are unsure about how to do any exercises, please consult a health professional or qualified personal trainer who can design a program specific to your sport.

Hip stability exercises

We cannot do core exercises without considering the hip muscles. Research has shown that the stability muscles likely to be weak are the quadratus femoris and the deep gluteals (see Figure 19 below).

If you place your hands on the outside of each hip, you will feel the muscles that run between these two bony prominences. All of them contribute to the stability of the hips and lower back.

Should you experience hip or buttock pain, be sure to include these hip and gluteal exercises in your daily exercise routine.

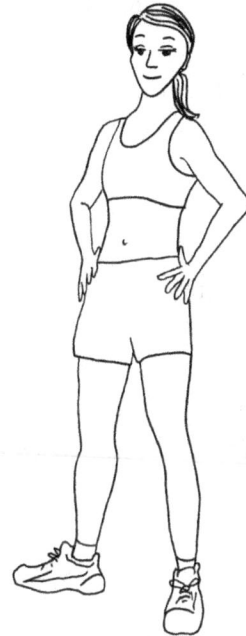

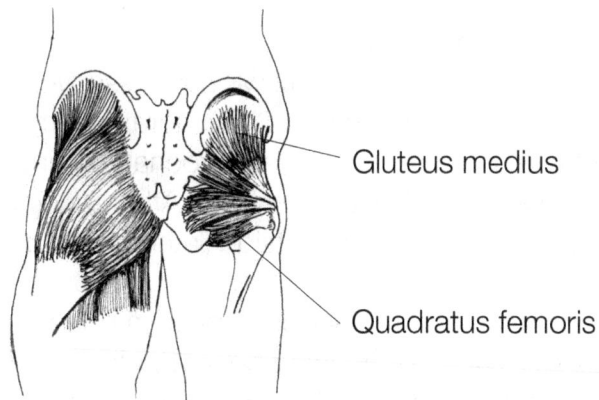

Gluteus medius

Quadratus femoris

Figure 19. The deep hip stability muscles include quadratus femoris and gluteus medius

📖 *Notes from the clinic*

Does your back ache when you stand?

Pain in the gluteals (buttocks) or on either side of the hips might be referred from the back, or due to weakness of the deep hip stabilising muscles.

Doing hip stability exercises can often reduce this postural fatigue. It might also settle any pain you experience on the outside of either hip.

Improving your stance will enable the deep hip muscles to engage a little more automatically.

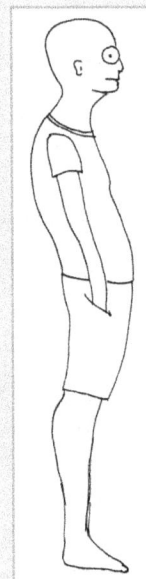

Exercise 25. Quadratus femoris

This exercise can help you strengthen a weaker gluteal muscle if you detect an imbalance between the two sides. You will have discovered this when you were doing the prone knee bend (Exercise 22). Quadratus femoris runs between the bone on the outside of the hip (the greater trochanter) and what we commonly call the sitting bones (the ischial tuberosities). After engaging quadratus femoris, you can often ease an ache on the outside (lateral) area of your hip.

Lying on your side with your knees flexed, place a pillow between your knees. Place your fingers between your sitting bone and the greater trochanter. You will feel a bit of a hollow there. Position your hand as if you were on the point of lifting your buttock muscle. Tap your foot to see whether you feel any contraction under your fingers. Sometimes tapping can wake this muscle up. Keep doing this for about 30 seconds and repeat six to eight times. This is called an isometric contraction of this muscle.

If you cannot feel any contraction when you tap your foot, draw your thigh towards your hip. At the same time, push your heels gently together. Then think of slightly lifting the top knee off the lower knee. Initiate the movement but do not lift the thigh. You should be able to feel activation in the muscle that is between the greater trochanter and the ischial tuberosity (the quadratus femoris). Hold this contraction for five to ten seconds and repeat four or five times.

If you find this exercise challenging, a physiotherapist can use Real time Ultrasound to teach you the correct way to engage the muscle. If you are uncertain about whether you are doing it correctly, I suggest moving on to the following gluteals-bridging exercise, which also engages the quadratus femoris muscle.

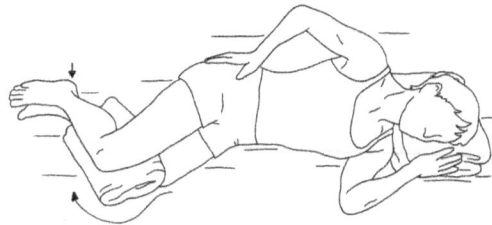

Exercise 26. Gluteals-bridging

Lying on your back with knees bent, imagine a ribbon between the bony prominences on the outside of the hips and think of drawing it a little tighter in the middle. Also draw the sitting bones together without over-tensing your gluteals. Breathe in; as you exhale, lift your pelvis off the ground. Hold for six to ten seconds; relax onto the floor again. Repeat eight to ten times.

Progression: When you find this exercise has become too easy, progress to keeping the hips off the ground and do eight to ten mini bottom lifts. That is, do not return your hips to the floor between each lift.

⚠ **CAUTION:** Do not over-extend your spine in either version of this exercise.

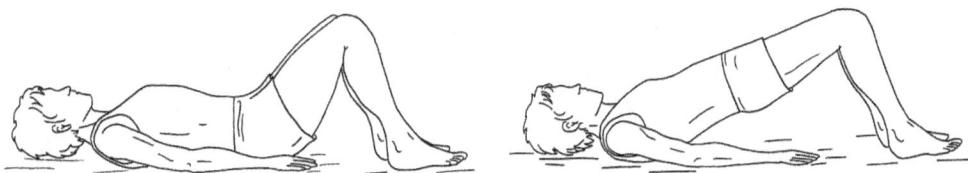

Exercise 27. Advanced gluteal and hip strengthening

Lying on your side, keep the lower leg straight and drop the knee of the top leg onto the ground. Shorten your thigh bone (femur) and raise the top leg so that it is horizontal to the ground. Hold for six to ten seconds and repeat four or five times. This is an advanced deep-hip stabilising exercise. If you find this exercise difficult, stay with the gluteal strengthening exercises with bridging.

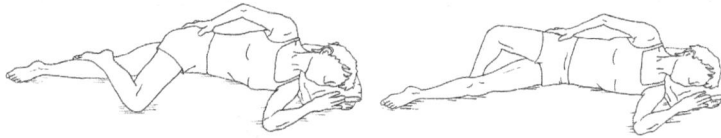

Activating the core muscles and gluteals

Once you can easily do the Level 1 and Level 2 stability exercises, engage the core while doing more functional movements. You are also ready to add fun exercises to challenge yourself a little more.

Exercise 28. Stability with squats; stand to sit

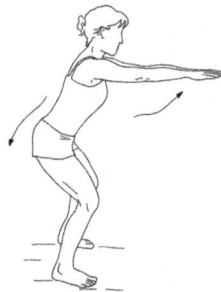

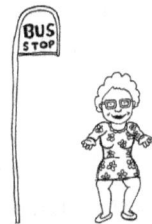

With feet apart, initiate the movement as if you were going to sit on a chair, then pretend that the chair is no longer there (do not let anyone take the chair away) and stand up again. Raise your arms to the front to help maintain your balance. Breathe in as you go to sit down; breathe out as you stand. Repeat this a few times during the day if you have a sedentary job; it is an excellent way to take some pressure off your back. You can even do small mini-movements like this when you are standing during the day. Make the movement so small that it is not visible to anyone around you, for instance at the bus stop or while you are standing in a queue. The smaller the movement the less you will need to use your arms for balance.

Advanced stability

Exercise 29. Hip flexion to extension

In front of a mirror, hug one knee to the chest, maintaining stability on the leg you are standing on. Now counter-resist the knee and the hands (that is, press knee and hands against each other) to engage the mid-back muscles. Keep your elbows bent. Once you feel stable, slowly extend the leg behind you. Repeat six to eight times with each leg. If you get too wobbly, stop and start the exercise again.

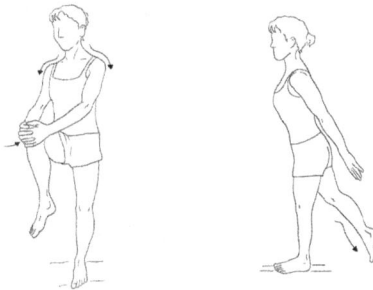

Exercise 30. Stork

Stand in front of a mirror; if possible, hold one foot and place it on the inside of the opposite thigh. Keep the foot lower if you cannot maintain stability at thigh level. Engage the gluteal muscles to maintain your upright posture and keep the hip in line; that is, do not drop into the hip as you do this. Extend your arms outwards at 90 degrees to the body. Try to keep breathing comfortably as you hold this position; maintaining it for a minute will be challenging.

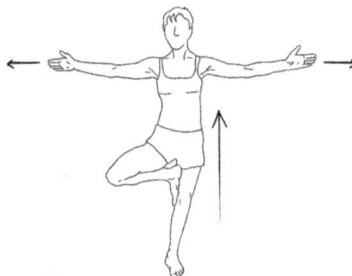

Exercise 31. Squat into hip extension

From a balanced standing position, place your palms together and then cross one leg over the other. Bring your ankle to 90 degrees and drop your knee as low as you can. Maintain your balance as you take your leg out and behind you. The goal is to maintain this position for one minute and repeat three or four times on each side.

Progression: Do the exercise with just the pads of the fingers pressed together; try to keep the pelvis parallel to the ground.

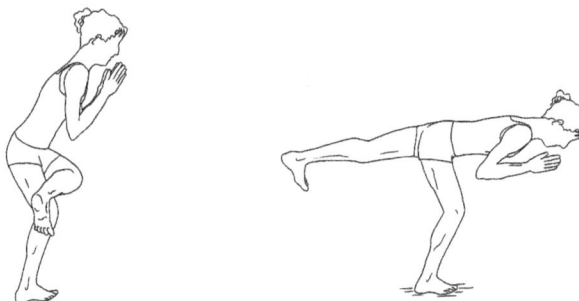

SUMMARY OF CORE EXERCISES

Level 1: Lying supine plus flutter and arm raise

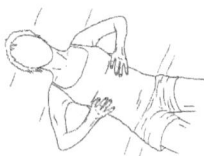

9

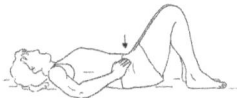

10

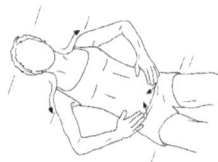

11

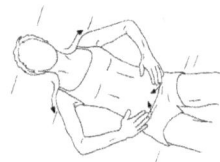

12

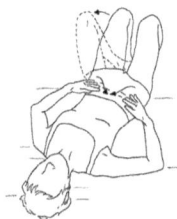

13

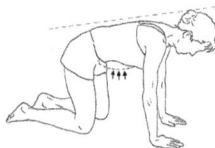

14

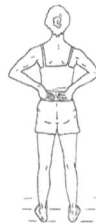

15

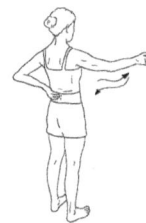

16

Stability progressions

Level 2: Supine stability using the arms and legs

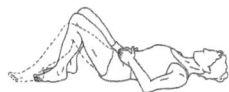

17

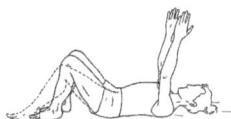

18

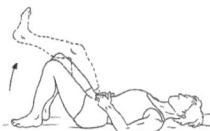

19

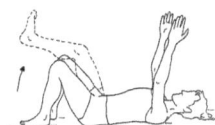

20

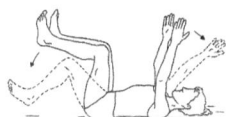

21

Prone stability

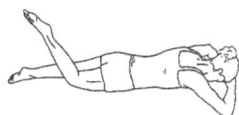

22

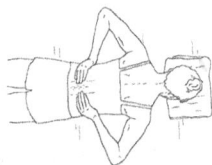

23

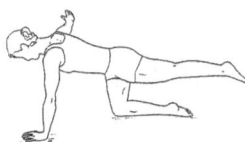

24

Hip stability

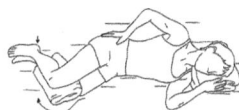

25

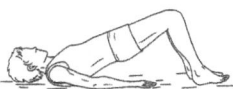

26

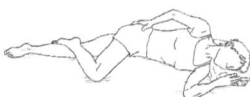

27

Intermediate stability and strengthening

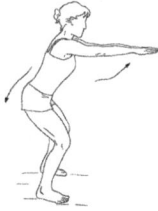 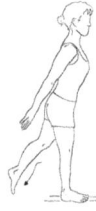 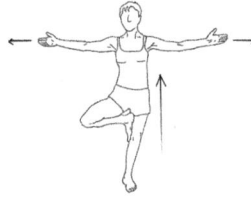 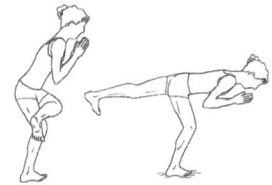

| 28 | 29 | 30 | 31 |

💡 Points to remember

▸ Start with basic exercises while lying down, to locate and engage your core muscles. Start by breathing more deeply into the diaphragm; engage the pelvic floor muscles, then the deep lower abdominal muscles, including transverse abdominus.

▸ Progress to engaging the core muscles when standing. Doing a small postural sway movement will activate them and adding a flutter movement of the hand or a repetitive movement of the arm will prompt the core muscles.

▸ Once you have mastered these basics, keep the core engaged as you progress to moving your arms and legs.

▸ Hip exercises are a vital part of core training. Include all of the stability exercises in your daily program; also do them while standing, to challenge the body.

✓≡ Actions to take

Spend about 10 to 15 minutes each day doing core exercises. The goal is to train these muscles so that they engage and thereby protect your back automatically, whether you are walking, sitting, lifting or doing other movements.

"Maybe I do need to start these core exercises - the little ones really are getting quite heavy when I take them for a walk"

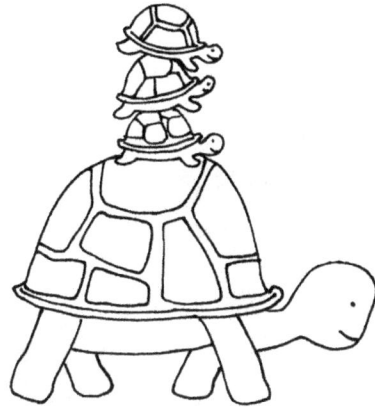

✏️ **Notes**

7 Stretching the back, hips and legs

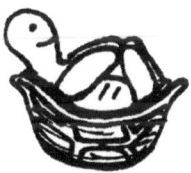

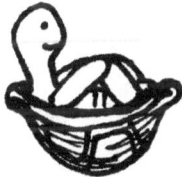

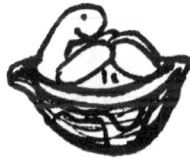

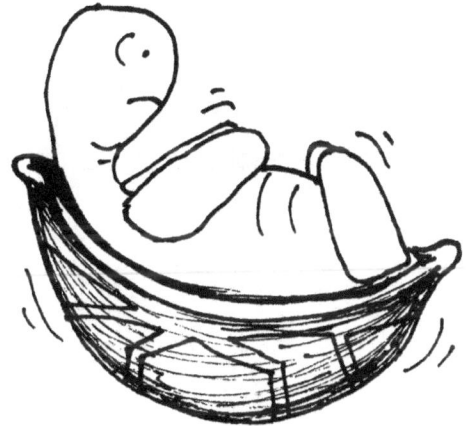

"How on earth can I stretch my hips and legs if I
can't even reach my belly button?"

Stability and neural exercises are just part of the solution. If you have a strong core but still feel stiff in all your joints, it is time to stretch. Muscles adapt and shorten with habitual use. You develop individual posture and work habits, whether your job is sedentary or entails heavy lifting. As well, leisure activities often add to muscle tightness. Think for a minute about how you use your phone or your tablet, or how you sit as you watch TV.

The superficial phasic muscles tend to adapt to our poor postural or work habits. In our legs, this means the hip flexors, gluteals, adductors, hamstrings and calf muscles; and in the back, the erector spinae. In this chapter you will learn how to stretch these muscles. In the following chapter you will learn how to stretch your neck, shoulders and mid back, and practise strengthening the muscles of your upper body.

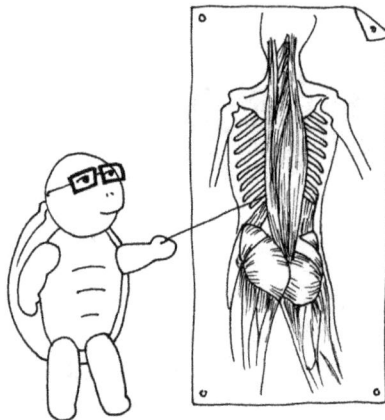

"Erector spinae is in the back and the gluteals are in the hips - who remembers?"

Helpful stretching tips

Stretching should feel good. The goal is to move gently into the position of a stretch, hold it for six to ten seconds, ease off, then move a little further into it again. Repeat this sequence two or three times at first. Eventually you will learn which stretches feel most helpful for your back, but do keep trying the more challenging stretches. Keep these points in mind:

▸ Even when stretching your hips and legs, relax your neck and shoulders.

▸ Keep breathing as you work into the stretch. It is so easy to accidently hold your breath, but this only makes your muscles tighten up more.

▸ Stretch when you are a little warmer, for instance after a walk or following a warm shower. It is crucial to warm up before you stretch.

Various sports cause different muscles to tighten up. You will find it helpful, between the times when you play your favourite sport, to focus on the muscles that are used the most in that sport.

For example, if you swim regularly, the pectorals and shoulder muscles will tighten. If you jog, the calf, hamstring and hip muscles will require particular attention.

LOWER BACK AND HIP STRETCHES

Exercise 32. Single leg hug for the hip

Lying on your back, hug one knee to your chest. Gently push the knee away from your body for five to ten seconds while pressing with the hands. Start with both knees bent the first few times you do this exercise. Progress to extending the other leg while you hug the knee to the chest. Relax; repeat four or five times with each leg.

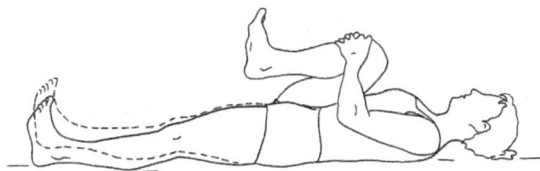

Exercise 33. Lower back release

Progress from the single leg hug; bring both knees to your chest. Counter-resist with the hands and knees for six to ten seconds. Repeat four or five times. Doing this exercise should feel great on the lower back; do not repeat the exercise if it does not.

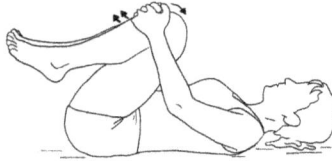

Exercise 34. Back arches and release

Now, on all fours, curve your back up as you breathe in. Do not hold the position; follow immediately with gentle curving of the back down towards the floor as you exhale. Return the spine to a more natural position, half-way between arching up or down, and gently take your hips back as you extend your arms in front. You will need to place your knees a little wider to achieve this with ease. You might also need to place a pillow between your waistline and thighs when you first start doing this stretch. Hold for 20 to 40 seconds; the stretch should feel relaxing and comfortable for your lower back.

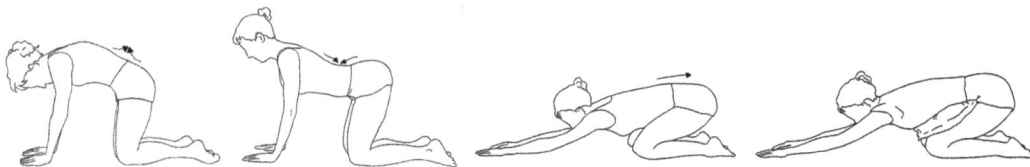

Exercise 35. Back extension

Lie face down, hands under your shoulders; gently use your arms to raise your head and shoulders. Rise first onto the elbows and then move into a full arch if you are experiencing no pain. Draw your lower abdominals in gently so that you are not locking into extension without any support for the lower back. Do not hold this extended position for longer than two or three seconds, as it is a dynamic movement. Repeat six to eight times.

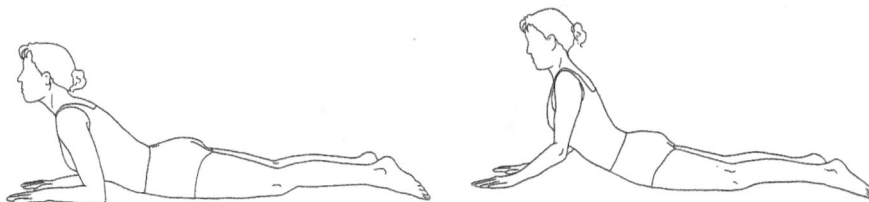

⚠ **CAUTION:** This exercise is not suitable for all back conditions. If you are especially flexible and feel vulnerable in the back even when you are only up on your elbows, or if you get pain in this extension position, please stop immediately.

An alternative to back extension exercises

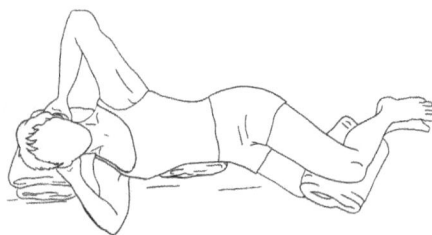

To maintain flexibility into extension, try doing back extension while lying on your side (see Exercise 4, above, for neck, arm and mid back stretch).

Standing back extension

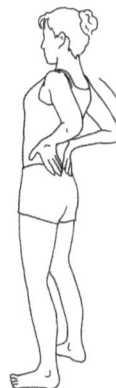

Another way to do a back arch, if extending while lying face down or on your side does not feel comfortable, is to extend while standing. Use your hands to support the small of your back and do two or three back arches. If you have a sedentary job, this is a beneficial exercise to do during regular breaks.

Exercise 36. Gentle spinal and hip rotation

Lie on your back with both knees bent, feet on the ground, arms outstretched at shoulder height. Let your knees roll to the floor in one direction as you hold the opposite shoulder on the ground. Repeat three or four times on each side.

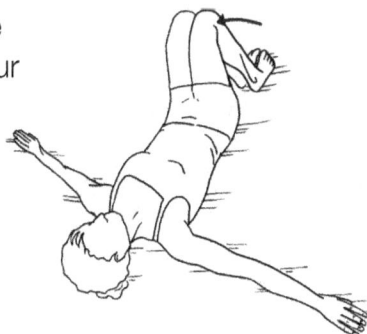

Exercise 37. Spinal rotation using a gym ball

If your back feels slightly unsupported or vulnerable when you do the previous exercise, lie on the ground with your lower legs atop a gym ball and do a very gentle rotation. Only let the legs fall to approximately 30 degrees from vertical, to left and right. This should feel relaxing for your lower back. You will also feel your core muscles activating when you are doing this exercise.

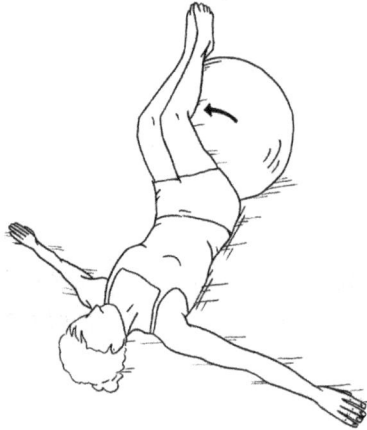

Exercise 38. Advanced hip and spinal rotation

⚠ **CAUTION:** Do not do this stretch if you have been diagnosed with an acute disc problem or your back is locked. This might aggravate your pain.

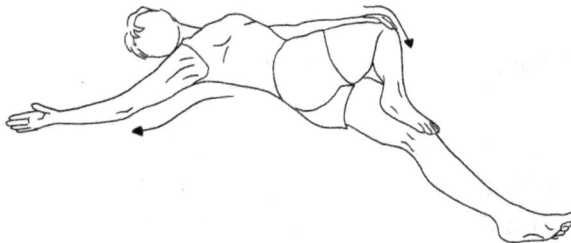

Lying on your back, take your right leg across your body. Place your left hand on your right knee to stretch it to the floor. Keep the right arm outstretched to improve the effectiveness of the stretch. Repeat on the other side.

Notes from the clinic

Do not click your back

"When I lie on my back and do spinal rotation I get a very audible click and my back feels so much better. Even when I simply stretch I get lots of clicks"

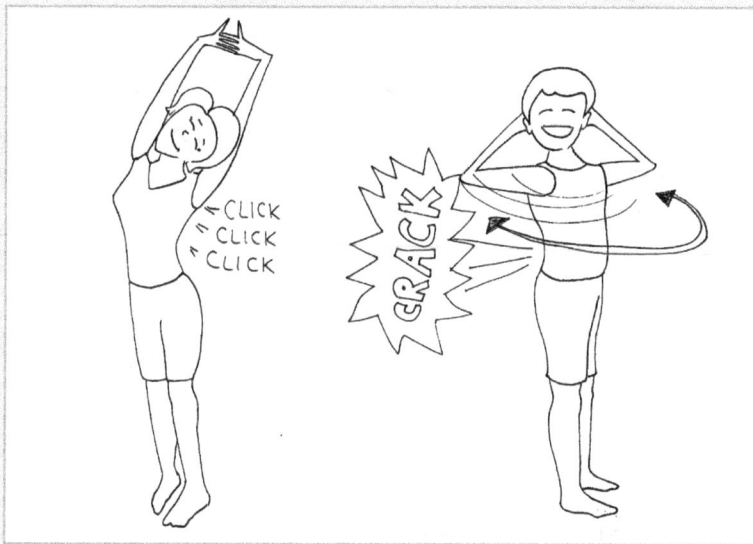

Do not deliberately click your back. When you stretch, expect audible clicks. If you are already highly flexible (hypermobile) you may get clicking without even intentionally trying to cause this. However, you must not manipulate your neck or back to make them click. Even though this might give you temporary relief from tight muscles or from pain it is likely you are releasing a joint that is already weak and unstable. You also might be straining or overstretching the ligaments at a specific level of your spine. This means that your body will simply tighten up again a few hours later.

The solution is to stretch and relax the superficial tight muscles and strengthen the weak ones. This will avert the need to click your own neck or back.

If you are especially flexible, you might be hypermobile.

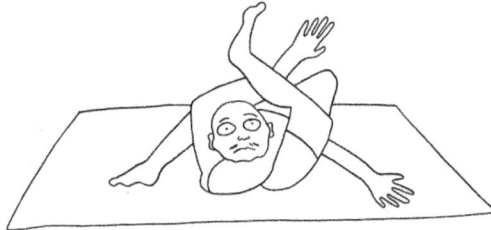

We all have variable flexibility in our muscles and joints. Some people can easily put their hands flat on the floor when they lean forward and others people can only get to their knees. It is possible to be highly flexible in all of your joints; this is called being hypermobile.

Can you:

▶ bend your thumb back onto your wrist

▶ hyper-extend your elbows or knees, and

▶ place the palms of your hands on the floor when you bend forward?

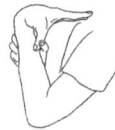

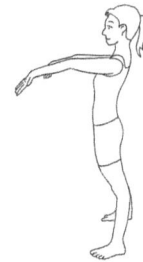

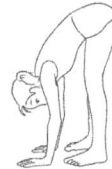

If you are able to do all these things, you are hypermobile.

This means that the focus of any exercise program you do needs to be on stability and strengthening. It is vital that you do not focus solely on stretching.

You can be hypermobile is some areas of your body and hypomobile (extremely stiff) in others. The most common postural pattern is hypermobility of the shoulders and hips, with stiffness in the mid-back. If this describes you, and you have back pain:

▸ start with core exercises

▸ combine them with stretches for your mid back, and

▸ focus on stability and strengthening for your shoulders and hips.

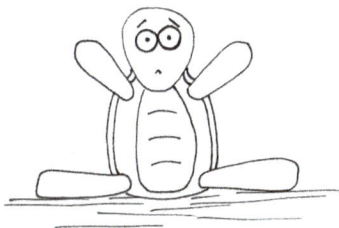

"Nope, definitely not hypermobile, this hurts"

HAMSTRINGS AND CALF STRETCHES

It is well known that tight hamstrings can cause back pain. When you bend over, or sit in a chair, tight hamstrings restrict the freedom and flexibility of the back and the hip muscles. The hamstrings come off the hip bones and insert below the knee, underneath the calf muscles. When the hamstrings are tight, often the calf muscles are too.

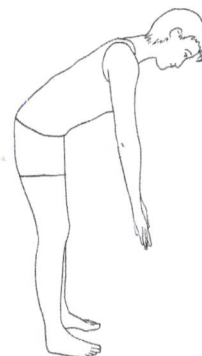

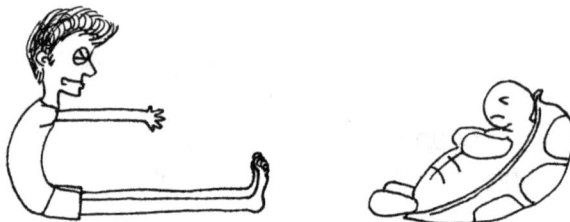

"Tight hamstrings might be causing my back pain"

Try these hamstring tests

⚠ **CAUTION:** Do neither of these tests if your back is sore.

Test 1: While sitting, see how far you can reach. You should be able to reach to your mid shin at least.

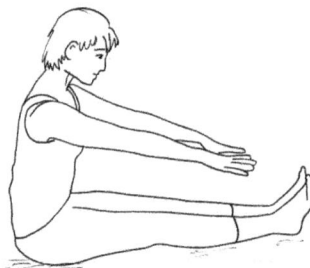

Test 2: While lying on your back, raise one leg. You should be able to take your leg approximately 70 to 90 degrees off the floor while the other leg is bent. If you cannot, tight hamstrings are probably contributing to your back pain. Be sure to include the following hamstring stretches in your daily exercise regime.

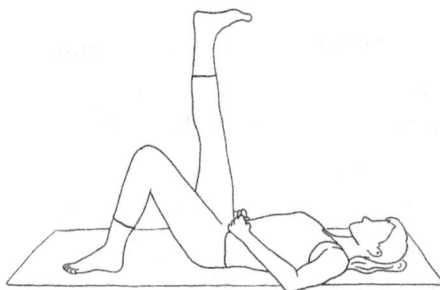

Exercise 39. Gentle hamstring stretch

Hug one thigh to your chest with your hands behind the thigh. Almost straighten the knee. Pull the ankle and toes back towards you; this will loosen the calf muscles and increase the effectiveness of the stretch. Bend and straighten the knee by a few degrees, two or three times, and this will start to loosen your hamstrings.

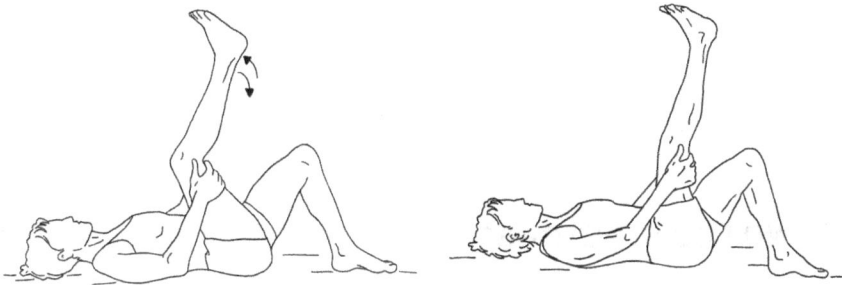

When you are sitting for extended periods of time, just extend one leg and try to straighten the knee while bringing the toes back towards you. This can be a great exercise to help stop your hamstrings from tightening up.

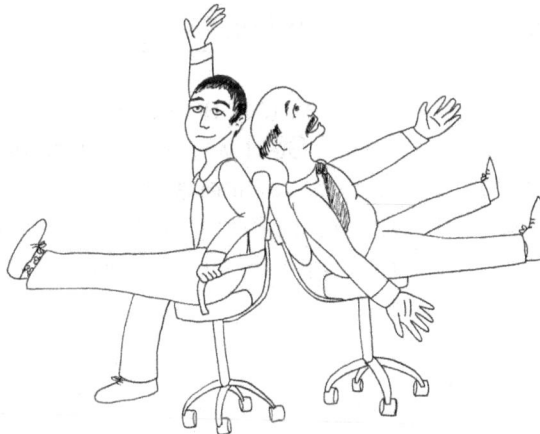

The correct way to stretch your hamstrings

If you have back pain, do not lie on your back and stretch your hamstrings with a straight knee, but keep the knee bent. Likewise, do not put your foot up on a table and lean forward with your knee straight trying to get your head onto your knee. Keep the knee bent in that posture as well. Both of these hamstring exercises, if done wrongly with knee straight, could potentially aggravate your back pain or the sciatic nerve. If you stretch a nerve in this sustained, static way, your back pain could return, about 30 minutes after stretching. This is called latent pain.

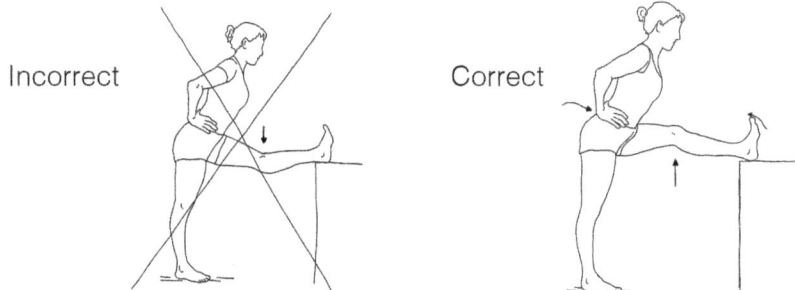

Incorrect   Correct

BACK, HIP AND LEG STRETCHES, INTERMEDIATE AND ADVANCED

The following stretches for your legs and hips are highly popular with clients who attend my regular physiotherapy classes. They are beneficial if you get hip or buttock pain. You will usually be able to engage your core more effectively after doing these hip and leg stretches.

Exercise 40. Advanced hamstring and calf stretch

Lie on a mat, place a towel around one foot and gradually pull the leg up towards the body, keeping it straight. Start with the opposite knee bent and progress to straightening that leg. You will feel a stretch in the calf muscle as well as the hamstring when you use a belt or towel. If you point the toes you will decrease the amount of calf stretch and feel it more in your hamstring. Relax the neck and shoulders as you do this stretch.

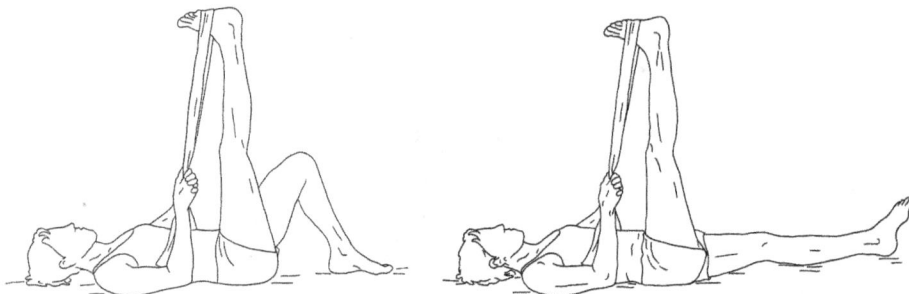

Exercise 41. Outer hip stretch

Place a towel or belt around one foot. Keep the knee of that leg slightly bent, and pull the foot across and upwards towards the opposite shoulder. You should feel a stretch in that buttock. Push the back of the hip down and into the floor to increase the effectiveness of the stretch. Keep the other leg bent and against a wall or in a doorway to keep the pelvis stable so that it does not roll to the side. Do this exercise on both sides.

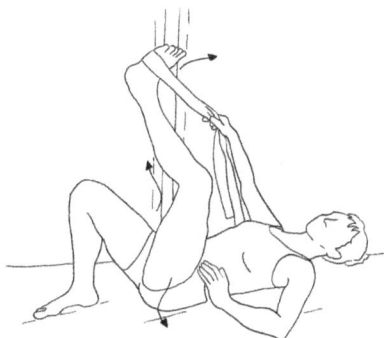

Notes from the clinic

Do not overstretch

You can avoid overstretching by knowing how flexible you are.

If you are already highly flexible, emphasise stability and strengthening rather than stretching.

A young man visited my physiotherapy clinic for his back pain. He was a builder. Each evening after work his back felt tight, so he would lie on his back and roll his legs right over his head. When I assessed him he could place his hands flat on the floor, indicating that he was hypermobile. The last thing he needed to do was to overstretch in the extreme flexion position he had been adopting. He and I discussed the sustained flexed positions he needed to do at his work. I showed him strengthening and stability exercises so he could work without needing to overstretch at the end of each day. After a few months, he broke the habit.

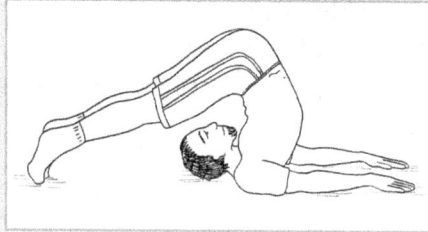

Stretching and flexibility for the adductors

Tight adductors are commonly associated with back pain. They could be tight because you have knees that turn inwards (internal rotation of the hips), or because of slightly over-pronated ("flat") feet, or the opposite, arches that are too high. Regularly sitting with one leg crossed over the other can be another cause of tightness in the adductors.

Try the following test to see whether you need to include adductor stretches in your regular back-care exercise regime.

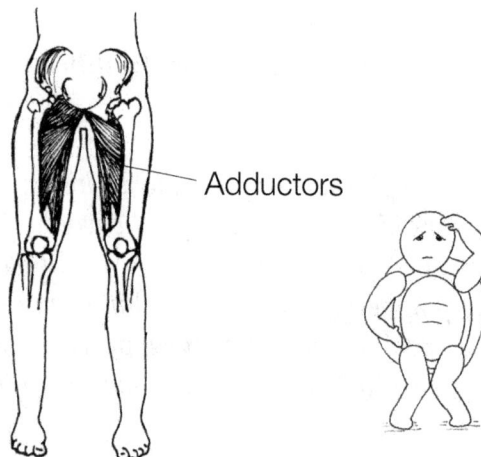

Adductors

Figure 20. Tight adductors might be contributing to your back pain

Exercise 42. Adductor flexibility test

You should be able to lie on your back and press the soles of your feet lightly together with your knees leaning outwards. If this is uncomfortable, rest your knees on pillows until it is easier to do.

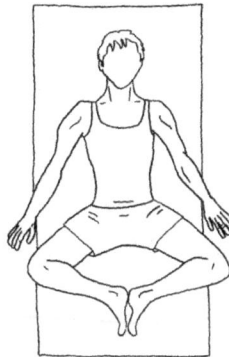

This is a relaxing exercise for the lower back as well as a test of your adductor flexibility.

Exercise 43. Adductor stretch while standing

Lean forward at the hips and place your elbows on a table. Bend one knee and drop into this side. You will feel a stretch in the inner thigh of your straight leg.

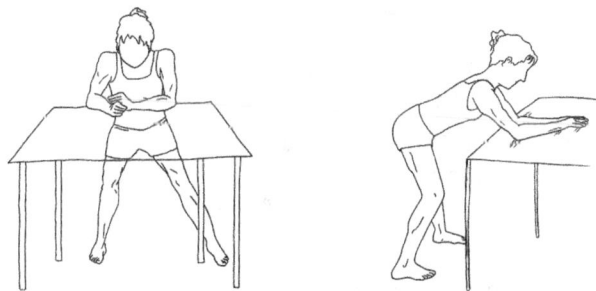

Exercise 44. Lying adductor stretch

Lie on a mat and place a band around one foot. With this knee bent, gently let the leg drop out to the side, using the band to support the leg. You will feel an inner thigh and upper hamstring stretch. Keep the other knee bent during this exercise.

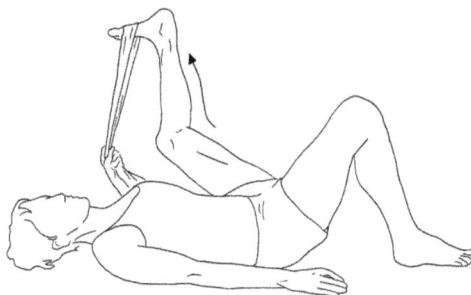

Exercise 45. Squat for advanced inner thigh stretch

Drop into a squat position. Grasp the inside of your ankles and rest your elbows against your knees. This is an excellent inner thigh stretch position, provided your knee and hip are sufficiently flexible to enable you to do it.

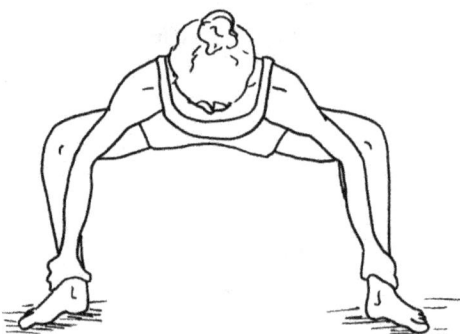

⚠ **CAUTION:** Do not do this exercise if you know you have weak pelvic floor muscles.

Exercise 46. Advanced hip, adductor, hamstring and calf stretch

Stand at right-angles to a wall and place one foot next to the wall. This will prevent slipping and enable you to concentrate on the places you are trying to stretch. Face your hips to the front, in the same direction as your head. Bend away from the wall, place the back of your hand against your shin bone and stretch the other arm upwards. Check that both arms are aligned. Do not let the top arm drop behind the body. Tuck in the chin and keep the head parallel to the ground. Stay in this position as you draw the shoulder-blades together and gently breathe into the diaphragm six to eight times. To challenge yourself a little more, work the hand down to your ankle. You might be able to put your hand on the ground but the aim is to maintain stability and not overstretch, so you usually do not need to do this.

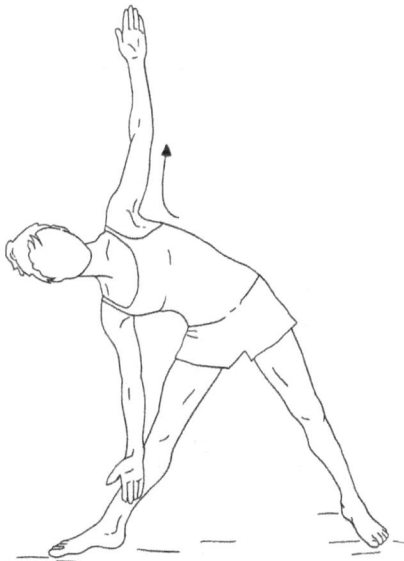

Stretching the hip flexors

Iliopsoas and rectus femoris are the two largest hip flexors. Tightness in either of these muscles can cause a forward (anterior) tilt of the pelvis, leading to excessive inward curving of the lumbar spine. This is called hyperlordosis and can cause the back muscles to tighten up.

Tight hip flexors can cause your back to ache after you have been standing for a long time. When standing, draw your stomach slightly inwards to reduce the curve in your back. This helps to relax your hip flexors.

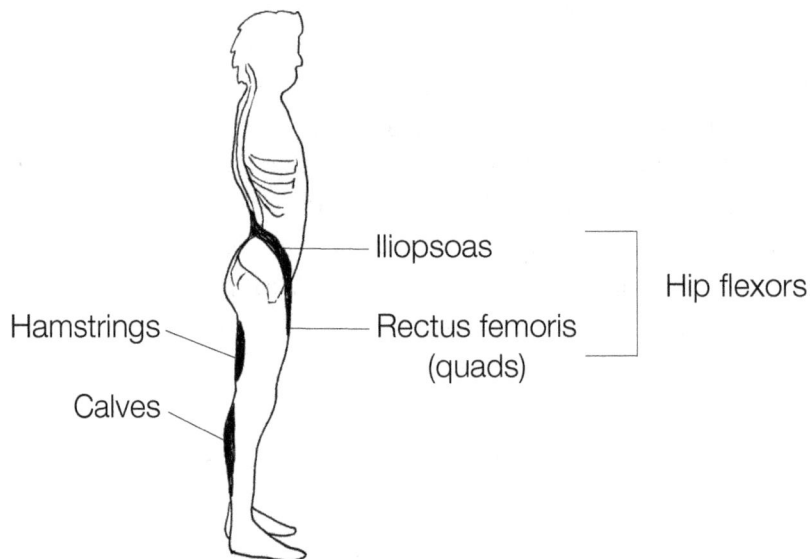

Figure 21: The hip flexors, iliopsoas and rectus femoris (quads)

Hip flexor stretches should help rectify an extra inward curve of your back and should ease any stiffness you feel in your hips or back when you stand after sitting for some time.

Exercise 47. Hip flexor stretch while standing

Stand up; take a step back with the right leg, placing it behind the left leg. Place your hand on the front of the right hip; this will help remind you to tuck the pelvis under and draw the abdomen in. Now lean the trunk slightly away from the right side. Push the feet away from each other lengthwise; tighten the buttock muscles and tuck the abdomen in even further for a more effective stretch. This is a stretch for the iliopsoas and other hip flexor muscles. Reverse leg positions to stretch the left leg.

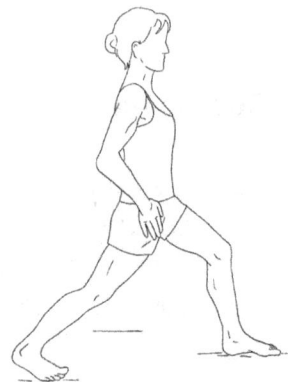

To make this exercise even more effective, take a bigger step. Hold for 15 to 30 seconds on each side.

Exercise 48. Hip flexor stretch using a chair or table

Place your foot on a chair or table behind you. If you need more stability, rest the whole of your knee and shin on the chair and use the back of the chair for balance. Tuck the pelvis under and inwards. Push the foot or shin into the chair. You should feel a stretch at the front of your thigh. You may need to bend the knee on your standing leg to improve the effectiveness of the stretch.

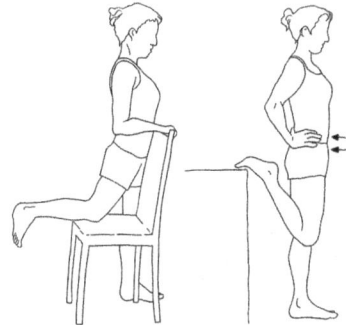

Exercise 49. Hip flexor stretch while kneeling

While kneeling on one knee, place one leg in front and lift the foot behind. If you do not feel balanced, place a small stool on one side to hold for more stability. Tuck the pelvis under and inwards until you feel a stretch at the front of the thigh of the back leg. Keep the spine straight, do not hyperextend (overarch) the back. Hold for 10 to 15 seconds; repeat on each side. If you cannot feel a stretch at the front of the thigh, place your back foot against a wall and you will feel it.

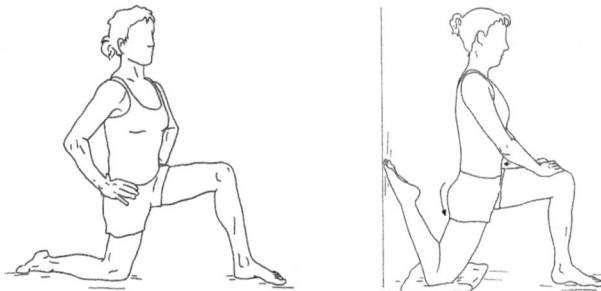

Do not hyperextend (overarch) your back when you are doing a hip flexor stretch; this can put too much pressure on your lower back and might cause pain.

Incorrect hip flexor stretch

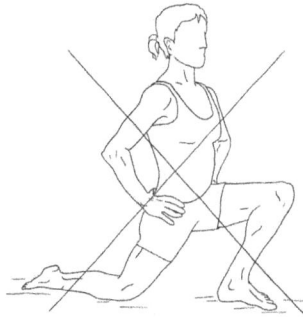

Exercise 50. Advanced hip and adductor release

Try this position if you did not feel any stretch at the front of the thigh in any of the above stretches. However, stop the stretch straight away if it is too stressful or you feel vulnerable in your lower back.

Lie face down; gently bend one leg and take it out to the side. Place your hand under the thigh of the bent leg and feel the gap where the front of the hip is off the ground. Now do this on the other side. Does it feel more or less tight? On the side that is tighter, that is, the one that is the highest off the ground, lie in this position and gently try to let the front of the thigh move closer to the ground. You can use your gluteals (buttock) muscles a little, but be very careful not to overarch and tighten your back muscles.

⚠ **CAUTION:** Do not do this exercise forcefully. It is a release exercise, so be gentle.

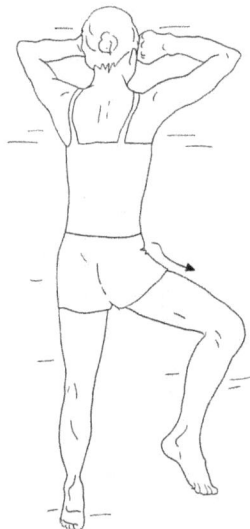

SUMMARY OF LOWER BACK, HIP AND LEG STRETCHES

Easy

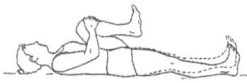

32

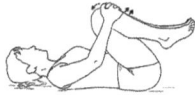

33

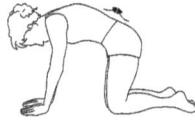

34

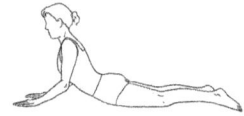

35

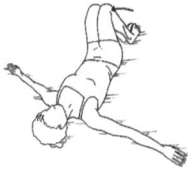

36

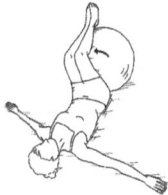

37

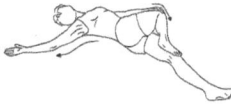

38

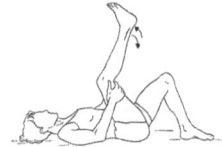

39

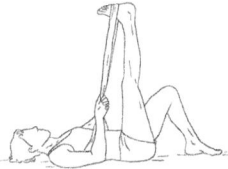

40

Intermediate and advanced

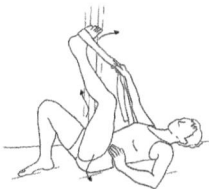

41

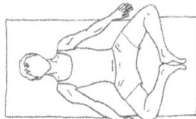

42

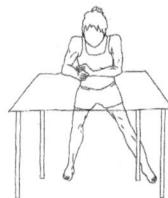

43

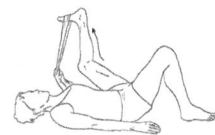

44

45   **46**   **47**   **48**

49   **50**

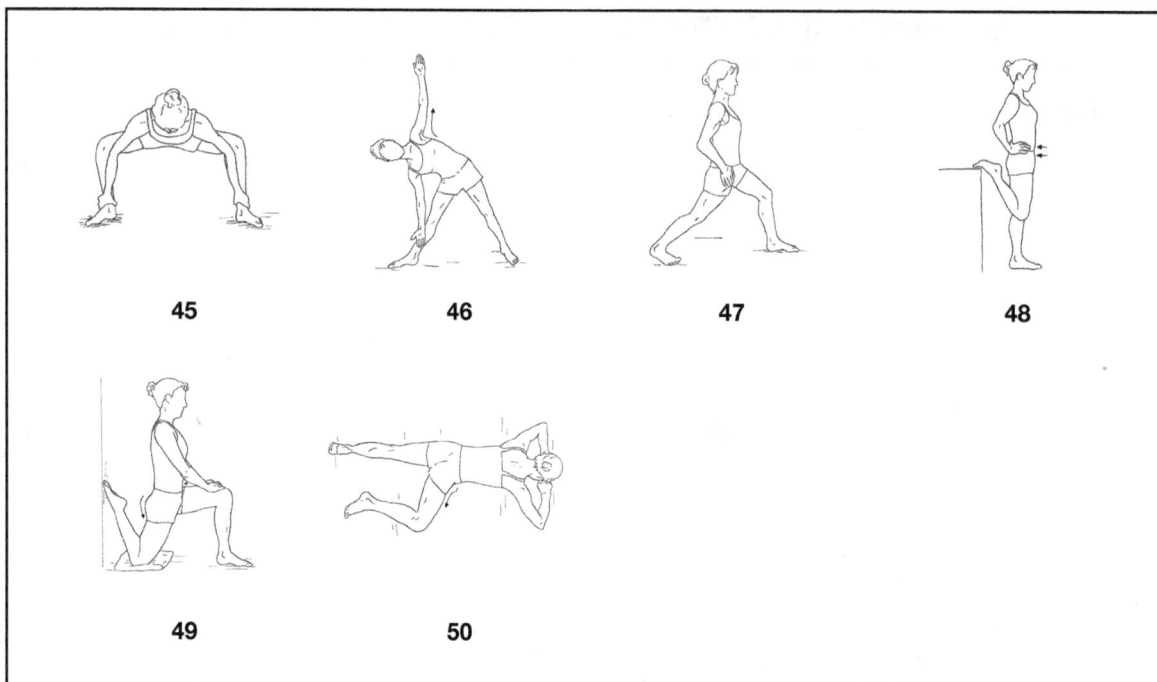

💡 **Points to remember**

▸ Tight muscles in the lower back, hip, hamstring, calves or adductors could be causing your back pain (or vice-versa).

▸ You have learned how to stretch safely; you know that you should stretch following exercise or after a warm shower.

▸ Neck and shoulders need to be relaxed, even when you are doing stretches for your back, hips and legs.

▸ Move gently into a stretch; hold for six to ten seconds; ease off the stretch position just a little for a few moments; then work into the stretch a little more. Do this two or three times for each stretch.

▸ If you are hypermobile, focus on stability and strengthening exercises; do not overdo the stretching.

✓= Actions to take

▸ Do the tests for hamstrings and adductors; find out whether you need to stretch those muscles.

▸ If you have an excessive inward curve of the lower back, add hip flexor stretches, which might ease your back pain.

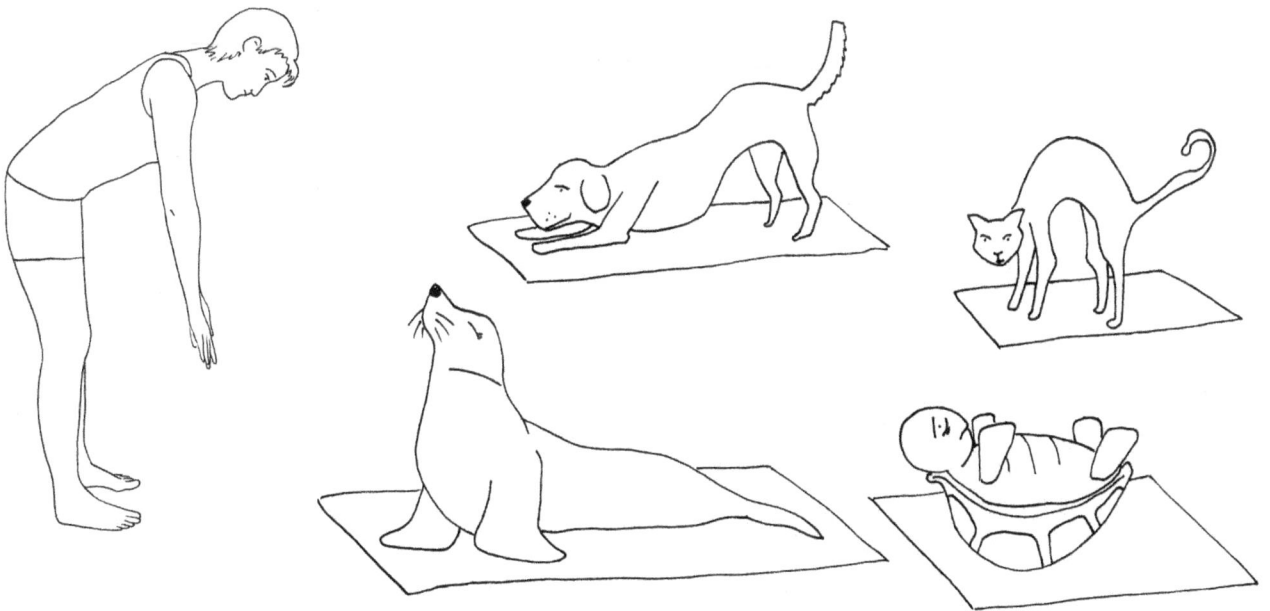

"Maybe I need longer arms?"

✏️ Notes

8 Stretching and stability for the neck, shoulders and mid back

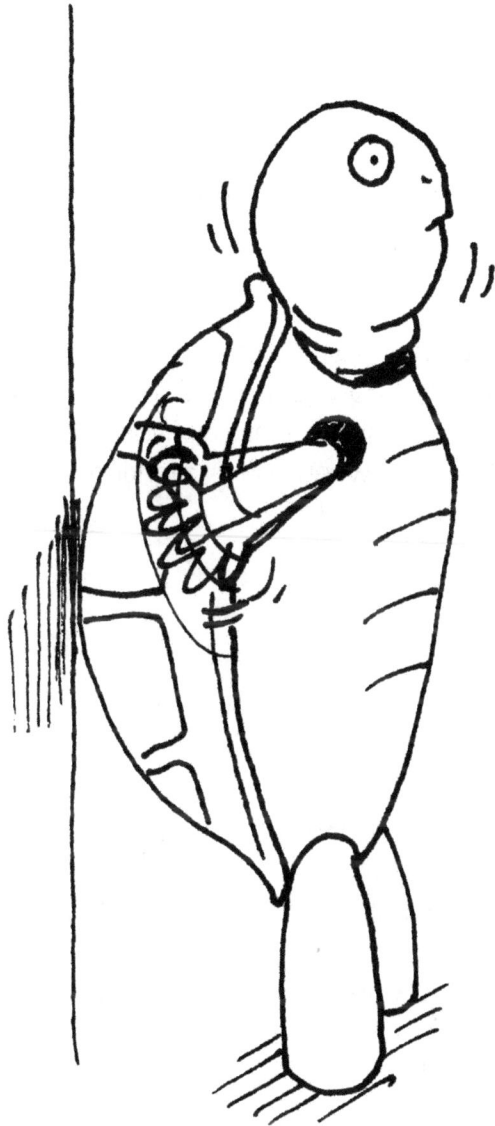

"I can't even get my head on the wall"

A forward head and neck position will cause tight neck and shoulder muscles, stiffness of the mid back and ultimately weak neck muscles. If you sit in this posture, you will breathe more shallowly and will quickly feel postural fatigue. This will make you slump even more. The result will be weak core muscles, which will produce even more stiffness of the mid and lower back.

Research has shown that the muscle imbalances occurring with neck pain or forward head and neck posture are similar to those that are associated with back pain. The superficial muscles tighten and the deep neck muscles weaken.

In this chapter you will learn how to relax the superficial tight muscles in neck and shoulders. You will find out how to retrain and activate the deep stabilising muscles. These exercises are highly beneficial if you experience neck pain or tightness in the upper shoulders when you sit working at the computer for long periods, as so many are obliged to do.

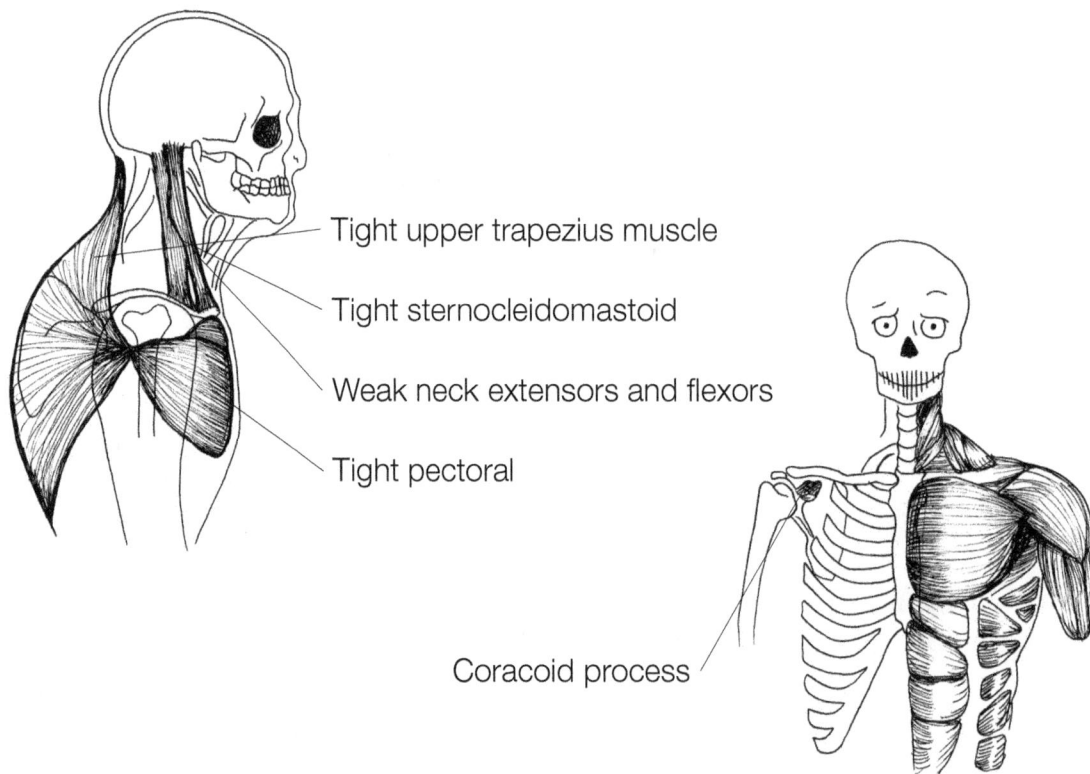

Tight upper trapezius muscle

Tight sternocleidomastoid

Weak neck extensors and flexors

Tight pectoral

Coracoid process

Figure 22. Muscles affected by poor head and neck posture

How poor posture influences core muscles

The phrenic nerve, which supplies the diaphragm, arises from the neck. The nerve supply for the transverse abdominus, the deep inner core muscle, comes from the thoracic spine. This means that a forward head and neck posture might constrict your breathing and a stiff mid back might prevent you from engaging the core effectively. Doing neural exercises and correcting your habitual head, neck and mid back posture will improve the automated action or engaging of the core muscles. These actions are likely to greatly reduce your lower back pain.

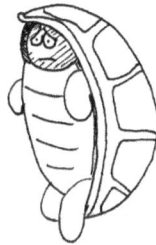

"Tucking my chin in and pulling my head in will help my core - wow - that's seriously amazing!

Exercise 51. Posture check for the neck, mid back and shoulders

▶ Try to stand with your back against a wall.

▶ Place your heels approximately six centimetres from the wall.

▶ Is the back of your head resting comfortably against the wall?

Place your fingers onto the front of the opposite shoulder. Slide your fingers off the ball and socket of the shoulder joint. Collapse into a slumped posture and you will easily feel a small bone called the coracoid process (see Figure 22). Now position your shoulders by drawing them back and down, and this bone will disappear. I call this "setting" the shoulders into a better posture.

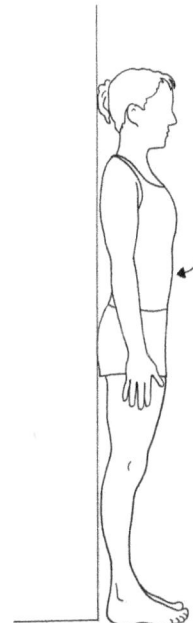

Ideally you should be able to rest the back of your head comfortably on the wall, and when you turn your arms outwards they should touch the wall.

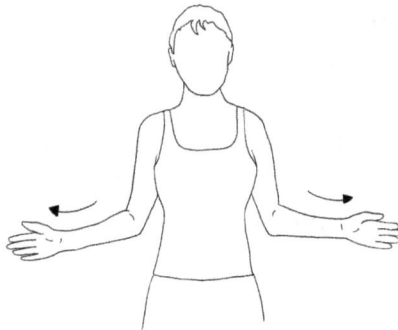

This is a beneficial exercise to do during the day to stretch the shoulders and mid back. If, when you tuck your chin in a little, you still cannot place the back of your head on the wall, place a small rolled up towel at the back of your head until this gets easier. In time you should not need the towel.

Exercise 52. Posture exercise

With your back against the wall, turn your arms outwards and stretch them up the wall. Repeat three or four times. Do this exercise when you need a break from working at the computer.

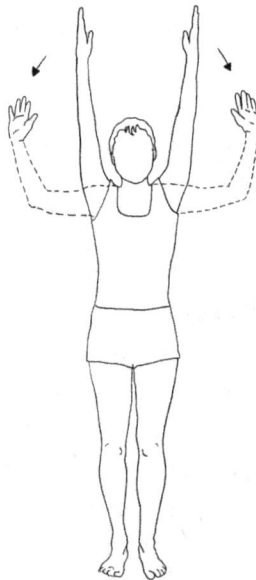

Treating tight muscles in the neck and shoulders

Before you do any strengthening exercises for the neck and mid back, locate the superficial tight muscles and relax them. The two muscles that tend to tighten are the sternocleidomastoid and the upper trapezius.

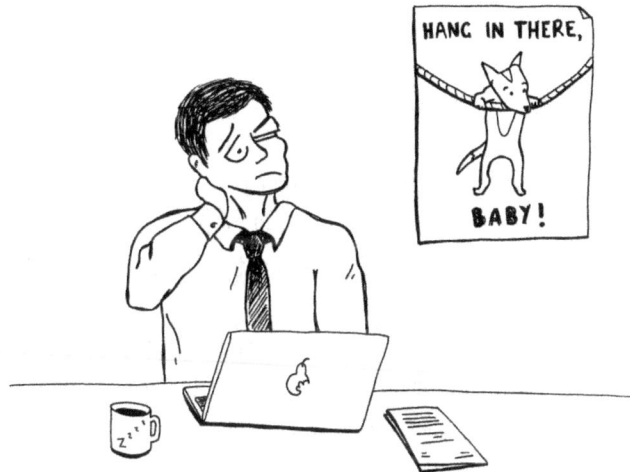

Exercise 53. Relaxing the sternocleidomastoid

Have a look in the mirror and tense your neck and shoulders. You will see a strap muscle that runs from the side of your neck to the front. This is the sternocleidomastoid. Place a hand on it and readjust head and neck until this muscle feels totally relaxed. You will probably find you need to tuck your chin in a little to achieve this. Do not exaggerate the movement. It needs to feel natural and comfortable.

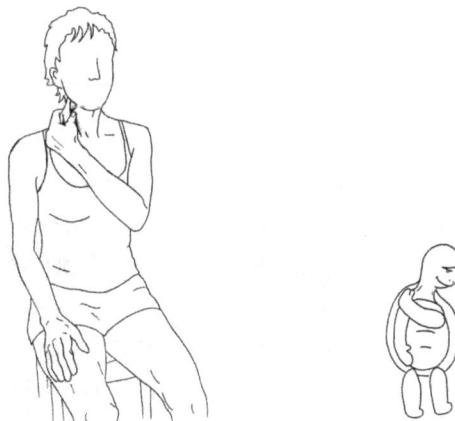

Exercise 54. Relaxing the upper trapezius

Place your left hand on top of your right shoulder, close to your neck. This is your upper trapezius muscle. Tighten it by shrugging your shoulder. Relax the muscle by altering the position of your shoulder. Feel with your left hand that the muscle is as relaxed as it can be. Repeat this exercise on the opposite side, using the right hand on the left shoulder.

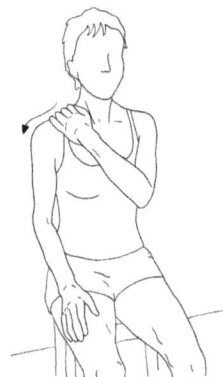

Once you have learned how to do this with your hand on your shoulder, you can consciously relax this muscle without needing to place your hand on it.

These exercises are valuable correctives to do during the day if you feel that that your neck and shoulders are tensing and you start to slump. You can also relax them when you are driving, but please only do this at the traffic lights and keep your hands on the steering wheel.

Once you have relaxed the tight muscles in your neck and shoulders, you are ready to do some stretches.

Exercise 55. Gentle neck stretch with hand over head

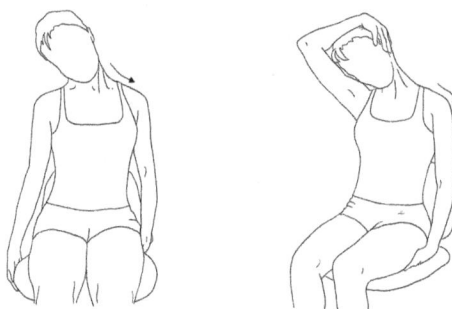

Sitting in a chair, place the left hand under the buttocks, palm facing upwards. Create a double chin by tucking your chin in, and tilt the head to the side, away from the hand you are sitting on. Pull the left shoulder downwards and bend that elbow. Then place the right hand over the head on the left ear and very gently stretch the neck. Keep altering the position of your head just a little until you find the ideal place that you can feel the stretch. Think of elongating the muscles on the left side of the neck, rather than pulling down on the head. Maintain for 10 to 15 seconds only. Return to the midline and stretch the other side. Repeat two or three times. Shrug the shoulders and relax them after doing this stretch.

Avoid incorrect neck stretching

It is important not to put your hand on your head and pull on it. This will aggravate any pain in your neck. To increase the effectiveness of stretching your neck muscles, lower the position of your shoulder instead of pulling on the head.

Notes from the clinic

Do not overstretch tight neck and shoulder muscles

A 38-year-old man was referred to me for treatment of his neck and lower back. He noticed that when he sat for a long time his right shoulder rolled forward and he could not keep it back. He had also noticed that when his neck and shoulders tightened his back would also tighten.

I looked at how he was working at his desk and found that he was using the mouse too far away from his body. He also needed to stop resting his chin in his hand while he was using the computer.

However, when I asked him to show me how he eased his neck pain, he placed his hand over the side of his head and stretched his neck so far over that his ear was on his shoulder. He also mentioned that each morning he did a rotation exercise and cracked his back before going to work.

His back was not going to settle down while he was doing these things. It is so important not to overstretch your neck in this way. You can stretch your neck much more effectively by tucking your chin in and simply tilting your head a little to one side. Then lower the shoulder on the same side that you are aiming to stretch, as opposed to pulling on your head.

It took this client a few months to break the habits of overstretching both his neck and his lower back. Once he achieved this goal and learned how to stretch and strengthen his back correctly, his postural aches and pains settled.

Exercise 56. Seated, stretching the base of the neck

Sit on the edge of a chair; cross the arms and put both hands around the outside of each knee. Pull back between the shoulder-blades and press the knees gently outwards. Stretch for 10 to 15 seconds and release. Repeat two or three times. To increase the intensity of the stretch, place your hands underneath the thighs and gently tilt your head a few degrees one way and then the other. You will feel the stretch at the base of the neck. Take care: you should feel relief, without aggravation of any neck pain.

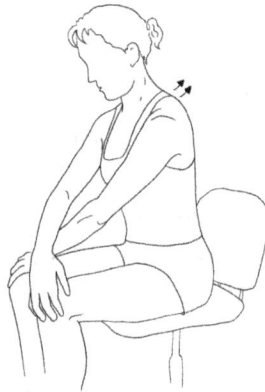

Exercise 57. Mid-back release, flexion and extension

Sit and place your hands on the outside of your thighs, close to your knees. Curve and stretch into the base of the neck and mid back. Shift your hands onto the inside of your thighs, close to your knees, and extend your spine.

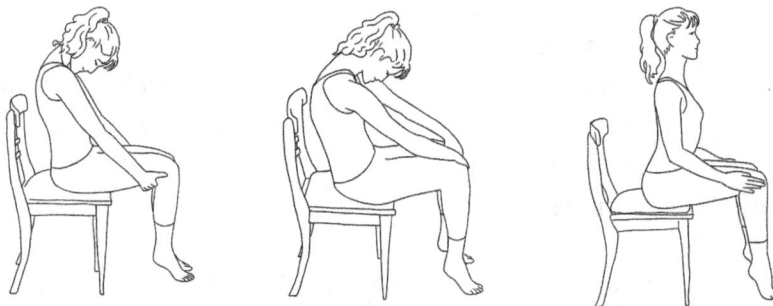

Exercise 58. Stretching the base of the neck, on the floor

Sit cross-legged on the floor; place your hands around the outside of your knees. Keep your spine quite straight and then let your knees move towards the ground as you stretch upwards and get a stretch at the base of the neck. Hold for six to ten seconds and release. Repeat two or three times. To increase the effectiveness of the stretch, tilt your head just slightly to one side, then the other.

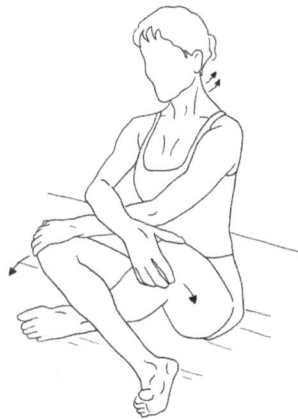

STABILITY EXERCISES FOR THE NECK

You are now ready to do some stability and strengthening exercises for the neck.

When you wake up in the morning does your head feel heavy? Do you find it really difficult to maintain good posture when you are sitting? Do you notice that your head keeps dropping forward and you end up in a slumped position? This may be because your neck stability muscles are weak. Can you believe that your head weighs from five to seven kilograms? Although you are not consciously thinking about them, there are stability muscles at the front and back of the neck, holding your head and neck in an ideal posture. Whenever you move your eyes to look at something, these muscles are pre-activated.

Research has shown that with neck pain there is a delayed reaction between using our eyes and the deep neck stability muscles. We take advantage of this automated connection to retrain these deep neck muscles, which in turn can improve overall head and neck posture.

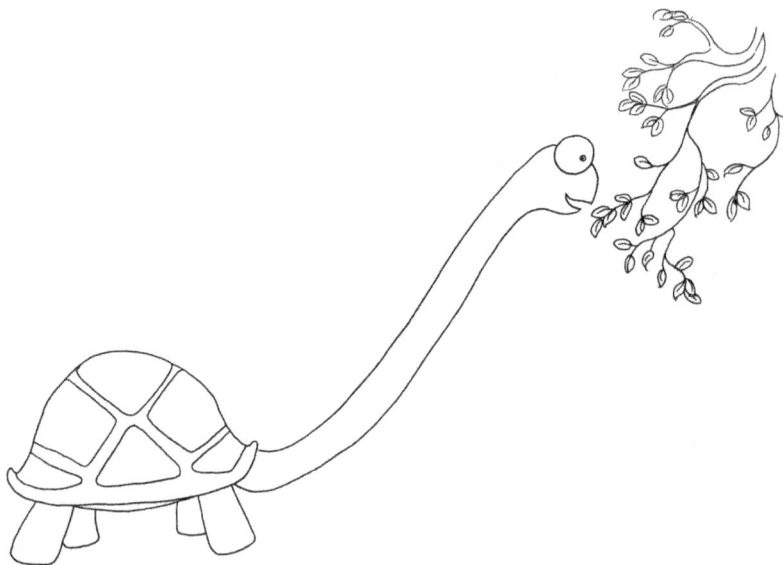

"Every time I use my eyes, my neck muscles are
engaged - that makes sense"

Exercise 59. Eye exercises that strengthen neck stability muscles

Follow this sequence:

▶ Sit on the edge of a chair.

▶ Place your fingers into the hollow area at either side at the top of your neck,
behind your head, at the base of your skull.

▶ Initiate the movement of beginning to stand up; then relax, but do not slump.

▶ Tuck the chin in slightly and push very gently into your fingers. You should
feel the muscles under your fingers engage.

▶ Now keep these muscles working as you take your eyes up. Hold for six to
ten seconds.

▶ Rest, then engage the muscles again as you take the eyes to the right, to the
left, and then up and down as if looking to the four corners of a wall (called
quadrants).

- Hold for six to ten seconds in each position and keep breathing as you maintain the small muscle contraction.

- If you cannot feel any muscle contraction, place one finger at the back of the head, push into it gently and keep your head in one position; do not move it. This gentle isometric contraction will activate the deep neck stability muscles.

- Reduce the intensity of the contraction and do the eye exercises again.

Once this exercise is easy to do, progress to this sequence:

- Take your eyes to the right, then turn your head to the right; return your eyes to the midline, then turn your head to the midline.

- Take your eyes to the left, then turn your head to the left; return your eyes to the midline, then turn your head to the midline.

- Next, carefully move your eyes up a little and follow with your head; return your eyes, then your head, to the midline.

- Now move your eyes down, followed by your head; next, move your eyes back to the midline, then move your head to the midline.

Once you have completed this exercise, shift your hands to the base of the neck and place your fingers on either side of the most prominent vertebra. Repeat the eye movements to each direction, including the quadrants, maintaining a gentle muscle contraction under your fingertips.

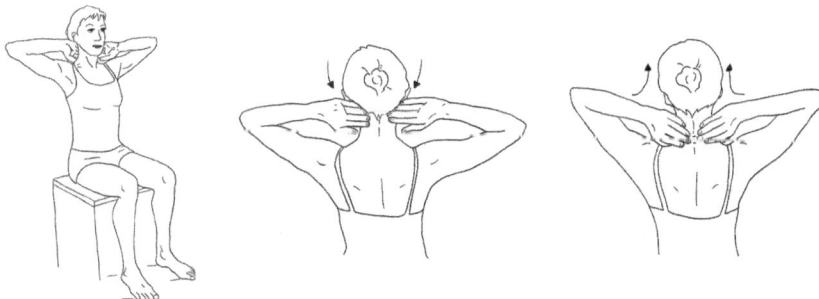

These eye and neck strengthening exercises are essential to improving your posture, and are particularly important if you have ever experienced a neck injury.

Exercise 60. Neck and neural mobility

Sit in a chair or stand up, with arms stretched out to the side. Look at one hand; extend your wrist upwards and move your arm slightly behind you. Continue to watch your hand. Extend and flex the wrist so that you are doing a neural exercise. (If you experience pins and needles in the fingers, stop this particular exercise and stay with the neck and eye exercises, keeping your head in the midline.) Repeat this movement on both sides.

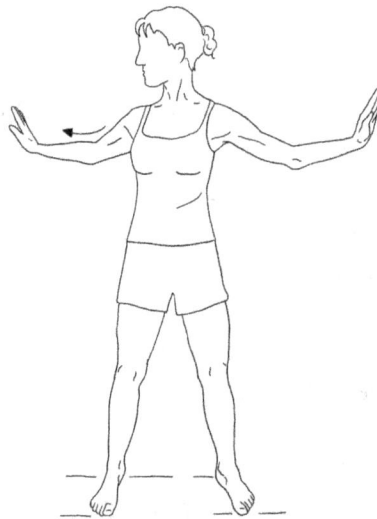

Exercise 61. Prone neck stability, engaging the deep neck extensors

If your head feels heavy when you do this exercise, this could indicate that your deep neck stability muscles at the back of your neck are weak.

Take great care not to lift your head off the ground. Instead, just think of lifting your head and initiate only a very small movement towards lifting your head.

Lie face down on the floor; place your hands under your forehead, palms down. Gently, pull your shoulder-blades back and downwards so that you are engaging the stability muscles between the shoulder-blades. This movement should be so minimal that if someone was watching you it would be barely discernible. Ask yourself, could you hold your shoulders in this position during the day? If the answer is no, you are overdoing it. Now, lengthen the back of the neck and think of lifting your head off the floor. Only start to initiate this movement; do not lift your head. Remember, the stability muscles engage when you even think you are about to move. This exercise is for activating the stability muscles at the back of the neck and in the mid-back. Hold for six to ten seconds and repeat two or three times. You will know that the muscles are stronger when your head no longer feels heavy.

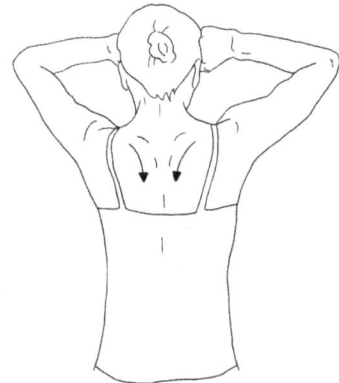

Exercise 62. Isometric neck strengthening for the deep neck flexors

Lie on your back with your knees bent and head resting on a rolled-up towel. Place your hands on the front of your neck on the sternocleidomastoid. Keep this muscle relaxed as you do a minor chin tuck and push the back of the head ever so gently into the towel for about six to ten seconds. Repeat two or three times. This should engage the deep neck flexors underneath the sternocleidomastoid, but if you feel this muscle tightening, you are overdoing it. Repeat the exercise with a little less pressure into the towel; continue to breathe while keeping this strong muscle relaxed.

Move your eyes in all eight directions, up, down, left, right and then quadrants, while you are pressing gently into the towel. This will improve the automated engagement of your deep neck stability muscles and reduce your postural fatigue, particularly if you need to work at the computer for long periods.

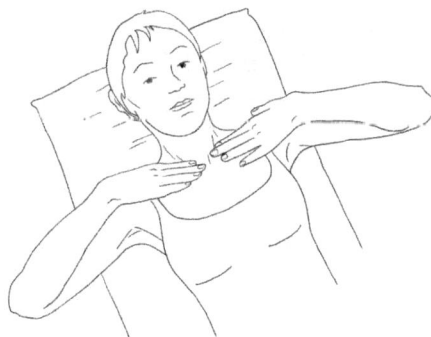

📖 *Notes from the clinic*

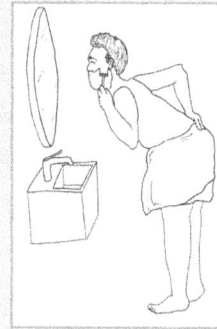

How strengthening neck muscles may resolve back pain

"I do push-ups, sit ups, planks and even have my own weights gym at home. But the moment I go to shave, my back feels so vulnerable – this makes me feel so old"

This patient was a fit-looking 190-centimetre (six-foot-four) man in his mid sixties. When I assessed his back, his erector spinae certainly appeared to be highly developed and strong, but he had a pronounced forward head and neck posture. I also noticed a scar on the back of his neck. He had forgotten to mention a rugby injury that had happened when he was 25 years old, for which he had needed neck surgery. I asked him whether he had ever done neck exercises. He said he had always tried to protect his neck and only did exercises for the rest of his body. I then got him to show me how he was doing his sit-ups, push-ups and a plank. He was doing all of the exercises with a forward head and neck posture, engaging no neck or abdominal core muscles. I started him with some eye and neck stability exercises, and then taught him how to strengthen and engage his core muscles without straining his neck. It took a few months, but when I last saw him, he had not had back pain for 12 months. This had been achieved by strengthening his neck muscles. He was much happier that he did not feel so old when he shaved.

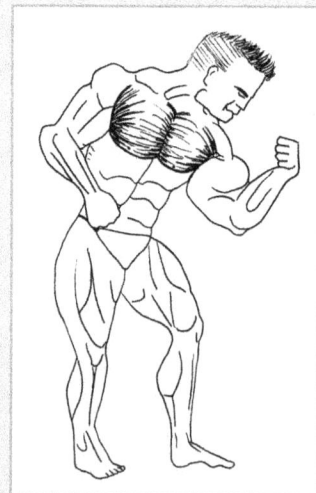

MID-BACK STRETCHES AND STRENGTHENING

Exercise 63. Pectoral stretching while standing

If you sit at a desk for much of the day, your upper shoulder muscles tighten, as do the muscles at the front of the chest, the pectorals. When you take a regular break from sitting, try this exercise.

Place a hand on a doorway or wall with the elbow at right-angles. Rotate the body away from the hand. Pull the shoulder-blade downwards and the humerus into the socket a little more. You will feel a stretch at the front of the shoulder.

Progress the exercise by moving the hand further up the wall and you will feel the muscles of the forearm being stretched too. Be careful not to twist the neck or body too much. Hold the stretch for 15 to 20 seconds. Repeat two or three times.

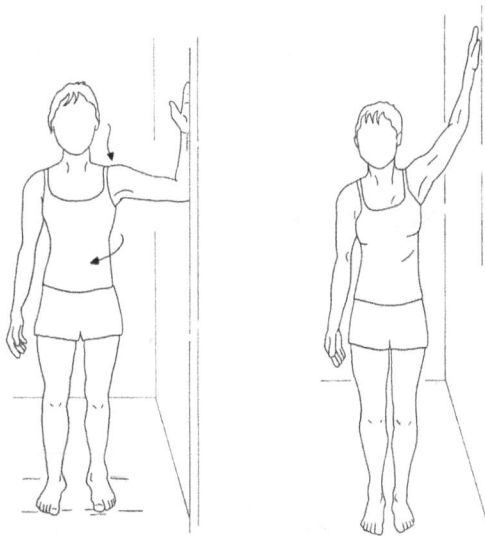

Exercise 64. Pectoral stretch, lying on your side

Lie on one side with your knees bent up and both arms stretched to the front. Raise the top arm up and over. Keep the elbow slightly bent and let the weight of gravity take it down and towards the floor. You should feel a stretch at the front of the shoulder all the way down to the fingers. Repeat two or three times with the head facing the front, then progress by letting your eyes and head follow as the hand is stretched behind you. Start this exercise with the elbow bent if it feels too intense with the arm straight (see Exercise 4 above).

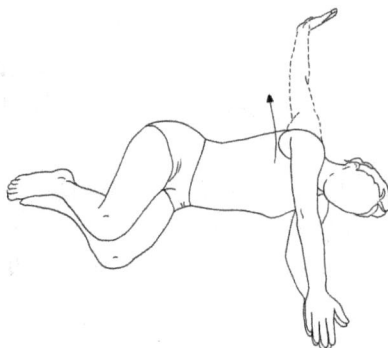

Exercise 65. Shoulder and mid-back stretch, threading the needle

On hands and knees, thread the right hand under and through to the left side of your body. Place the hand on the floor with palm up. Curve the spine upwards and draw into the right shoulder-blade. You should find a position where you can feel whether you have tight muscles under the shoulder blade, then feel them easing. If you cannot feel this, change the placement of your hand so that the stretch feels more effective to you. Push the back of the hand into the floor for six to ten seconds. Be sure to curve the back upwards. Repeat two or three times on each side of the body.

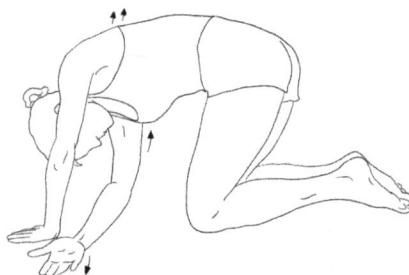

This exercise can provide you with a lot of relief if you experience tightness underneath or between the shoulder-blades.

Exercise 66. Intermediate shoulder and mid-back stretch

On hands and knees, slide one hand out to the front and draw it back, then slide the other hand out; extend the mid-back as you slide each hand forward. If you feel no pain, extend both hands together out to the front. Keep the hands turned upwards or extended. Work on pulling the shoulder-blades together and letting the mid-back move towards the floor. Hold for 15 to 30 seconds. You can also use a fitball to do this stretch.

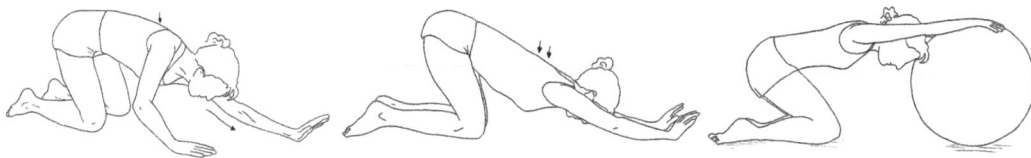

Exercise 67. Advanced mid-back side stretch

Stand at right-angles to a wall and place the palm of the closest hand onto the wall. Bring the other hand over your head and place the palm of this hand on the wall, so that the fingers of each hand are facing each other. Work with your breathing as you exhale gently and stretch into the shoulder and rib cage. If there is any pain in the lower back this is not an appropriate exercise for you.

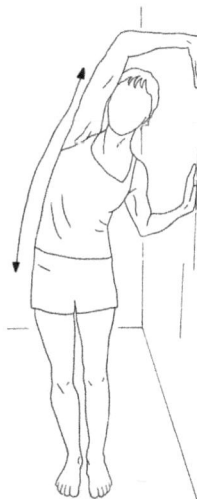

Exercise 68. Advanced mid-back and shoulder stretch

Sitting on the ground, stretch one leg out with the knee straight and bend the other leg so that your foot is next to your knee. Place a belt around the foot of the outstretched leg and hold the ends with the opposite hand. Place your other hand under the top arm and clasp the opposite knee. Turn your body so that you are looking under the top arm. Breathe in, and as you exhale keep the arm closest to the floor bent and keep elongating the side of your spine that is closest to the ceiling. You should feel this stretch anywhere from the mid back all the way down to the hip.

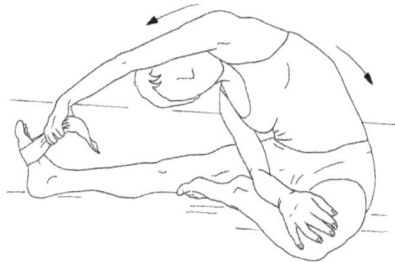

Exercise 69. Mid-back strengthening using a band

Hold one end of an elasticised band in each hand. Breathe in; as you exhale, gently turn each hand outwards a little, only about 15 to 20 degrees. Hold for five to eight seconds in this position as you breathe comfortably. This helps to activate some of the small stability muscles of the neck and mid back. Transfer your weight ever so slightly onto your heels and you will feel your core muscles working a little more.

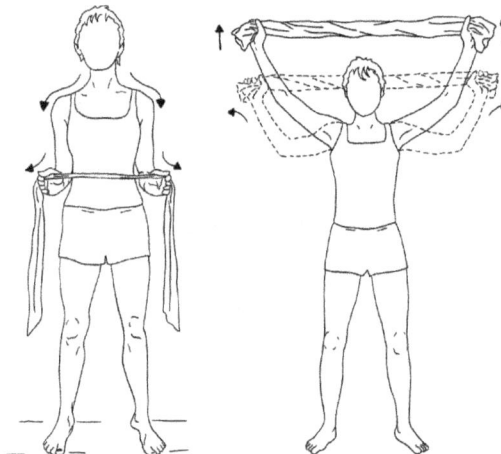

Progress this exercise by raising the band above your head. Keep the shoulder-blades down and towards the spine, and apply a gentle outward pull on the band. As you breathe out, pull the band behind the head. Return to the resting position and repeat the exercise four or five times.

Both of these exercises can be done using a rolled-up towel instead of an elasticised band.

Exercise 70. Mid-back strengthening while sitting

Place the elastic band around your mid back. Secure the ends of the band around each thumb. With thumbs facing up, pull the band outwards slightly and then take it out in front of you at a slight upwards angle. Control the band as you return to your starting position.

This exercise improves posture and increases your overall mid-back, shoulder and neck strength.

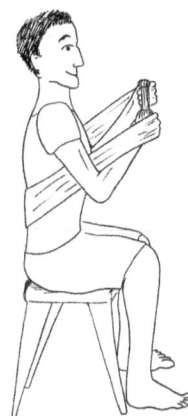

Exercise 71. Prone mid-back strengthening

Lie face-down with arms by your sides; create a double chin and raise your forehead and arms two or three millimetres off the floor. Keep the shoulder-blades pulled down towards the spine. Do not let the shoulders move upwards and towards the ears, or you will use the wrong muscles during the exercise. Hold for six to ten seconds and relax. Repeat four to six times. Try to hold the position and the contraction of the muscles a little longer, each time you raise your arms, until you can easily hold the position for 30 seconds. Pull the abdomen in slightly so that you do not arch your back as you do the exercise. Take care not to overarch, to avoid straining the lower back.

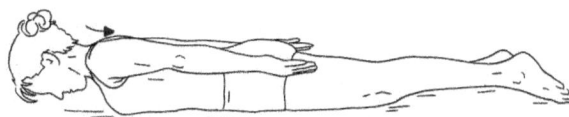

Exercise 72. Advanced mid-back strengthening

⚠️ **CAUTION:** Skip this exercise if an extension position aggravates your lower back pain.

Start with your feet shoulder-width apart and bend forward into a slight squat position. Without shifting the position of your feet, turn them both outwards to engage your gluteal muscles. Now raise your arms so that your elbows are next to your ears. Keep the thumbs facing up towards the ceiling. Breathe in; as you exhale, raise the arms a little higher. Tuck in the chin to protect the neck. To make the exercise more challenging, flex at the hips a little more but keep the arms straight and elbows next to the ears. There should be no pain in your lower back but you will feel the muscles in your mid back working. Try to maintain this position for 30 seconds to a minute. Repeat no more than once or twice.

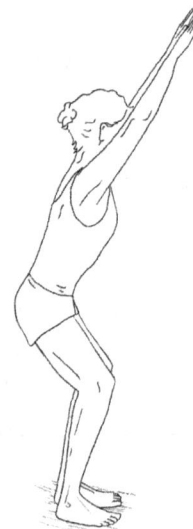

SUMMARY OF NECK, SHOULDER AND MID-BACK EXERCISES

Neck stretches

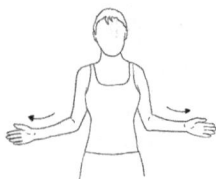

51

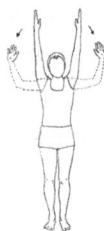

52

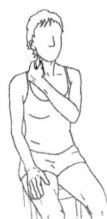

53

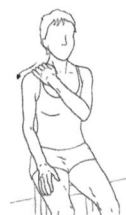

54

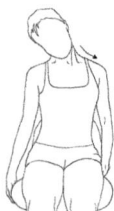

55

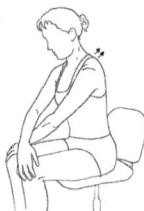

56

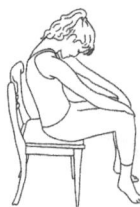

57

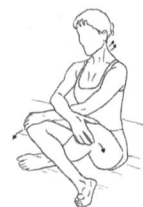

58

Neck stability

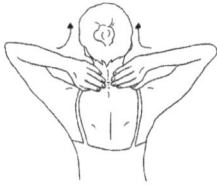

59

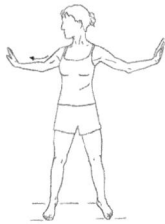

60

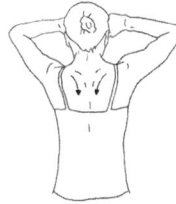

61

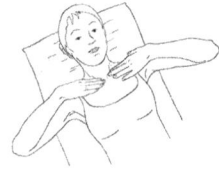

62

Mid-back stretches and strengthening

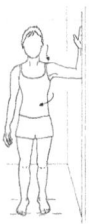

63

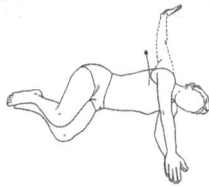

64

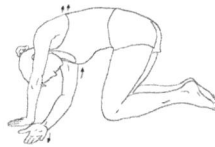

65

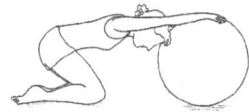

66

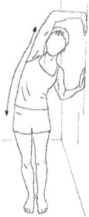

67

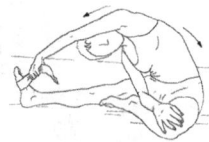

68

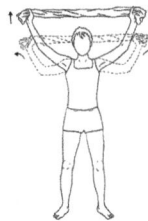

69

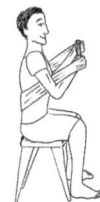

70

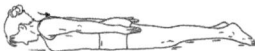

71

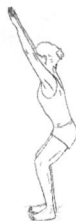

72

💡 Points to remember

▶ Overcoming back pain requires attention to neck, mid back and overall posture and strength.

▶ Forward head and neck posture might stop your core muscles from working automatically, which could contribute to your back pain.

▶ If you are feeling tight in neck and shoulders, place a hand on your upper shoulder or neck muscle and change your posture so that these muscles feel more relaxed. When you stand with your back against a wall, you should be able to outwardly rotate your arms so that the back of the arms can touch the wall. Do this exercise during the day if you sit for a long time.

▶ Use your eyes to activate the neck stability muscles; monitor the engagement of these muscles. This can reduce your neck pain and improve head and neck posture.

✓= Actions to take

Do a posture check at various times during the day, especially if you sit at the computer for a long time.

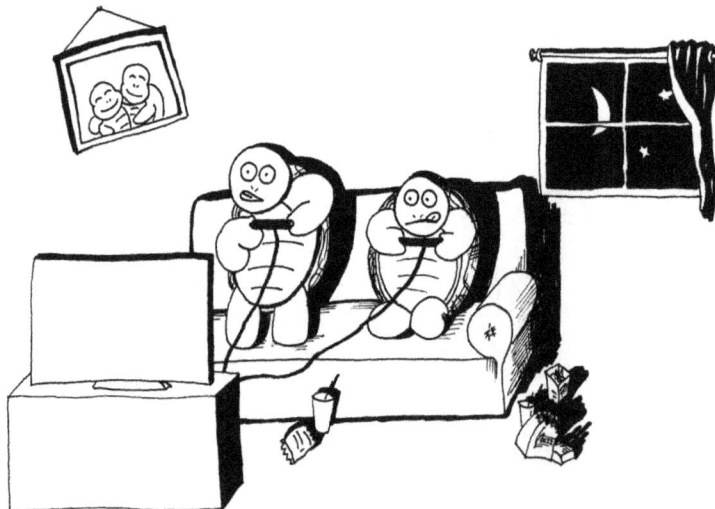

"How was your day dear?"
"Terrible. So tiring. I had to sit down all day."

Notes

9 Posture

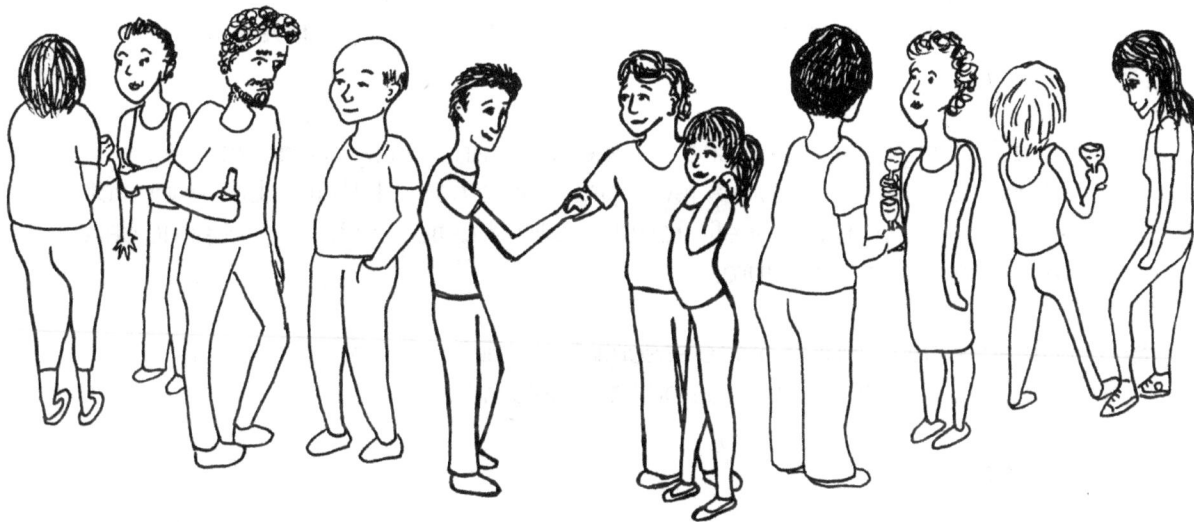

Knowing what you can and cannot change

Most of your poor postural habits can be improved with attention to daily habits and a little more self-awareness. However, some aspects of posture are hard to change. Your innate postural type can influence your inherent flexibility and strength, and vice-versa. Knowing more about your postural type can help you to know what areas you need to stretch and where you need to strengthen. This will also help you to select the exercises that most effectively relieve your back pain.

Review each postural type and see whether you can identify yours. You might find that you have features from a few types; this is normal. With a better idea of your postural type, you will benefit from the following tips on how to change daily habits and improve your posture.

Start with an understanding of the essential elements of good posture and the typical aspects of poor posture, as outlined below.

Ideal posture

Ideally, a line drawn through a profile of your body would run from the middle of your ear to just behind your ankle bone. This optimum alignment is challenged by your daily habits, but it can be achieved.

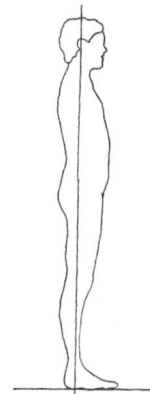

Have someone photograph you from the side; print the photograph and draw a vertical line through the printed profile. This is a simple way to find out where you need to stretch and what areas of your body you need to strengthen.

Typical poor posture

Bad postural habits can include:

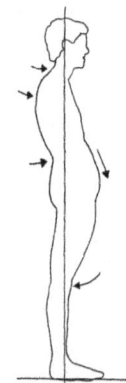

▸ forward head and neck

▸ stiff mid back

▶ weak lower abdominals, and

▶ knees locked back, causing tight calf muscles and hamstrings.

The wrong way to correct your posture

Over-correcting your posture by being too rigid is wrong. You will tire quickly and revert to poor posture within minutes.

Helpful quick tips to improve your posture

Below are some effective ways to counteract bad posture.

▶ Adjust your body so that you feel taller. Keep your neck and shoulders relaxed and gently engage your core muscles.

▶ Imagine a small torch resting on your chest-bone (sternum). Lift the torch up and outwards, as though shining it into the eyes of someone you were speaking to. Automatically, your head and neck will be in a better position and more balanced over your shoulders.

▶ Lift your body weight up and out of your pelvis. Gently engage your lower abdominals and draw them towards your spine without over tensing your upper abdominals and without holding your breath.

▶ Soften and slightly flex the knees. Stand on a gentle incline, about five centimetres higher at the front than the back. You should feel your core muscles engage and find it easier to correct your head and neck posture.

▶ If you are stiff in your mid back, rotate your hands outwards from the elbows, while sitting or standing. For an extra stretch, do this exercise against a wall (see Exercise 51, Chapter 8).

Be aware of and correct your posture at all times, whether you are sitting, standing or walking, and not only when someone is watching you.

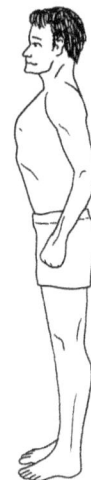

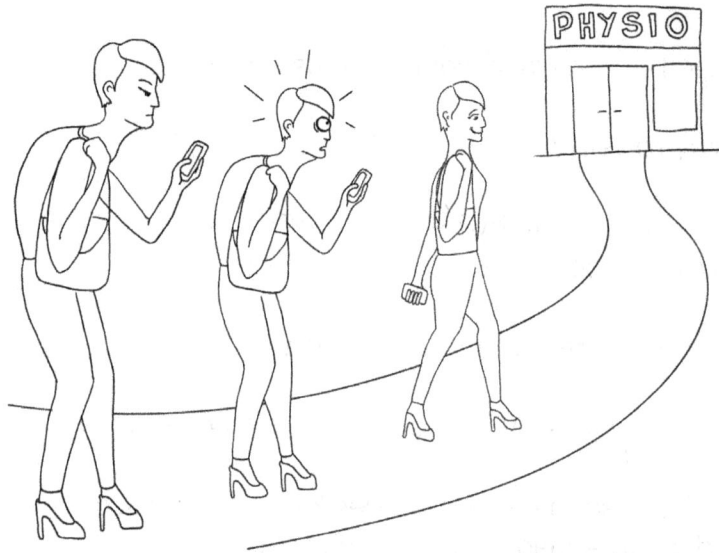

"But the physio said I had such good posture"

 Notes from the clinic

The benefits of 3D assessment

Three-dimensional (3D) postural assessment, until recently available only to athletes in sports science laboratories, can now be used in physiotherapy and other clinics. One of the benefits is immediate awareness of your posture. This type of assessment can also help monitor your technique in doing stability exercises such as the single leg stand, lunge and squat. Be sure to ask whether your health professional or personal trainer is using 3D technology.

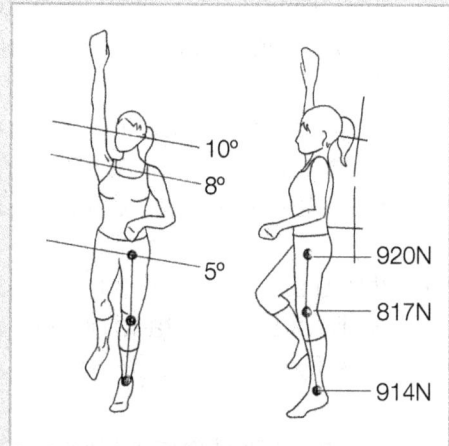

Typical postural types

Below are the features of the four most common postural types, with the key exercises for each. You can select the most appropriate ones to include in your exercise program.

1. HYPERKYPHOSIS

Defining feature

Hyperkyphosis comes from an excessively flexed position of the thoracic spine. It usually includes forward head and neck posture and tightness of the shoulders. An excessive inward curve or hyperlordosis of the lumbar spine is often associated with this postural type.

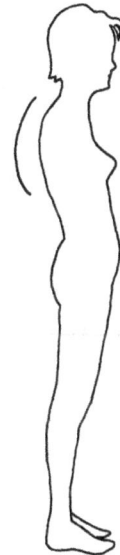

Specifics

Features of hyperkyphosis include:

▶ tight upper trapezius and superficial neck muscles (sternocleidomastoid) that need to be relaxed and stretched

▶ weak neck and mid-back extensors that need strengthening

▶ tight pectoral muscles needing to be stretched

▶ limited outward (external) shoulder rotation that needs stretching, and

▶ stiff thoracic spine, often reduced mid-back flexion and extension; needs to be stretched.

Postural tip

Shift your weight onto your heels fractionally, and think of lifting all of your body up and off your feet. Do not claw your toes. Imagine that you are increasing the distance across the front of the chest and looking a little further ahead, not downwards. Draw your shoulders gently back and down.

Thinking of "placing your shoulder-blades into their pockets" is a helpful cue.

SUGGESTED EXERCISES FOR HYPERKYPHOSIS

Relaxing the upper traps (Exercise 54, page 146)

Place your hand on your opposite shoulder. Now reposition your shoulder so that the upper neck and shoulder muscles feel more relaxed. You will need to tuck your chin in a little to achieve this. Repeat on both sides.

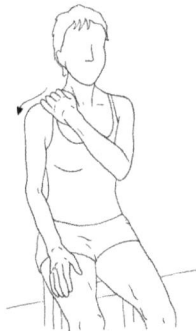

Shoulder rotation with back against a wall (Exercise 51, page 143)

Stand with your back against a wall. Outwardly rotate the hands, keeping your elbows close to your side and at 90 degrees. The goal of this exercise is to improve shoulder mobility as well as mid-back extension. Repeat the outward rotation of your arms two or three times. You can also do this easily when sitting in a chair.

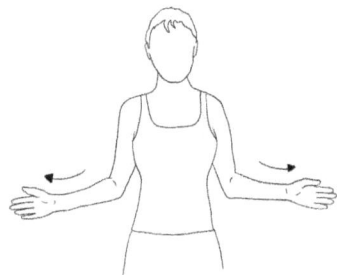

Pectoral stretch (Exercise 63, page 155)

Place your hand on a door frame, keeping your elbow at 90 degrees. Step through the doorway a little. The goal is to stretch the mid-back muscles, and the pectoral muscles at the front of the chest.

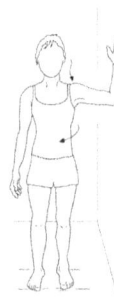

Activating the deep neck stability muscles (Exercise 59, page 150)

While sitting in a chair, place your hands behind your head and feel for the prominent vertebra at the base of the neck. Move as if you are about to stand up and you will feel the neck muscles engage under your fingers. Tuck the chin in a little and push the back of your head into your fingers for six to ten seconds. Repeat two or three times. Refer to Exercise 59 to learn how to use the eye muscles to activate the neck stability muscles even more effectively.

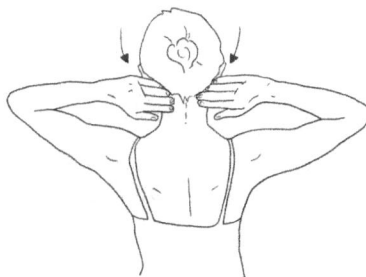

This is an excellent exercise if you become sore in your neck and shoulders when you sit for a long time.

Mid-back stretch while lying on your side (Exercise 64, page 156)

Lie on your side, extend your arms to the front and place your palms together. Now extend one arm above, across the body and behind you. Follow your hand with your eyes; this will allow your head to move comfortably as you stretch your arm. You may need to rest your head on a rolled-up towel or a pillow to do this exercise. The goal is to stretch your mid back and improve your shoulder flexibility.

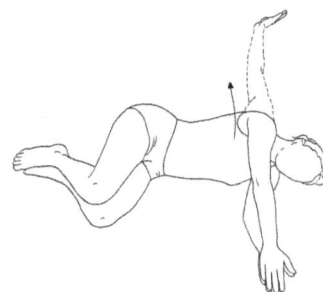

Four-point kneel and thoracic extension (Exercise 66, page 157)

While on your hands and knees, extend one hand in front of you. Keep the wrist extended to increase the effectiveness of the stretch.

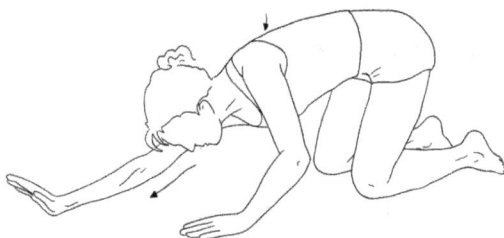

Mid-back stability with a towel or band (Exercise 69, page 158)

Hold each end of a towel and stretch it above your head. You should feel the stretch through your shoulders and mid back.

If your flexibility allows, stretch the towel down behind your head. This exercise is easier to do after a warm shower.

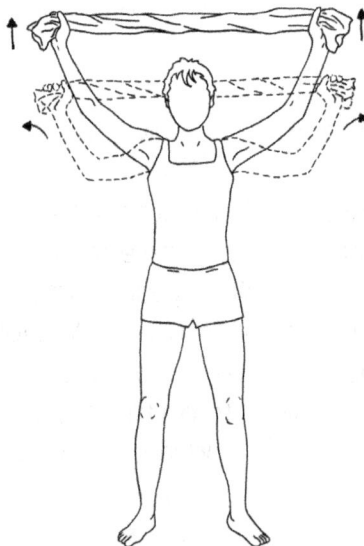

For mid-back strengthening, progress to using an elasticised band. Take the ends of the band and outwardly rotate it while keeping your elbows by your side. Control the movement as you return to the start position. Repeat six to eight times. Try Exercise 70 once you find Exercise 69 too easy (see page 159).

Mid-back stretches (Exercise 65, page 156)

After completing the mid-back strengthening, you will need to stretch the mid-back muscles. Starting on your hands and knees, place the right hand under and through to the left side. At the same time as you push the back of this hand into the floor, stretch your body upwards and across to the right. You should feel a stretch under your shoulder-blade. Repeat the same exercise with your left hand.

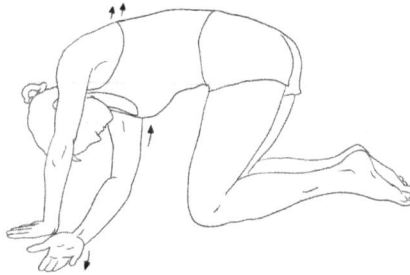

Deep neck extensor strengthening while prone (Exercise 61, page 152)

Lie face down and rest your forehead on the back of your hands. Relax the neck and shoulders, then gently draw them back and down. Engage the muscles at the back of your neck by lifting your head just a little off the ground (one or two millimetres only). This exercise activates the deep stabilising muscles of the neck and mid back. Maintain this slight lift of the head while you breathe four or five times. If possible do two or three sets.

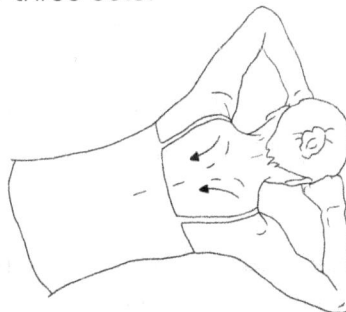

2. HYPERLORDOSIS

Defining feature

It is normal to have an inward curve of the lower back but with hyperlordosis the curve is exaggerated. This is usually associated with tight hip flexors and hamstrings, and weak lower abdominals.

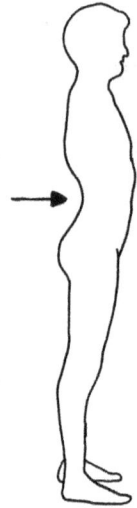

Specifics

Features of hyperlordosis include:

▸ tight superficial back extensors and hamstrings that need stretching

▸ anterior pelvic tilt associated with tight hip flexors (psoas, quadriceps or adductors; all of these muscles need to be relaxed or stretched), and

▸ weak lower abdominals that need strengthening.

Postural tip

Shift your weight onto your heels, soften and relax your back muscles and gently engage your lower abdominals.

Try these steps to achieve better posture. While standing, imagine someone very gently pushing you on the chest. You will feel your lower abdominals activate as you imagine you are stopping yourself from falling. Be aware of this gentle engagement of your lower abdominals during the day. Another small movement is to draw your belly button towards your spine, but do not over-tense or brace your abdominal muscles.

Place your hands in the small of your back and soften your back muscles when you stand. Place your hand on your hip flexors when you are sitting, and try to relax them as much as possible.

Place your feet over a chair and totally relax your hip flexors and adductors; this will also help your lower-back muscles to relax.

SUGGESTED EXERCISES FOR HYPERLORDOSIS

Postural sway (Exercise 15, page 98)

Place your hands around and onto your lower back. Gently
draw your lower abdominals inwards so that you can reduce the
inward curve of your lower back. Do a minimal sway movement
onto your heels and this will help you find a position where your
lower-back muscles feel more relaxed.

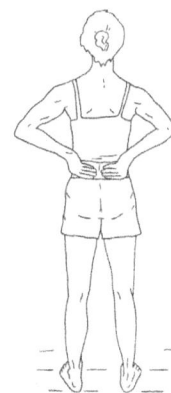

Relaxing the lower back and hip flexors (Exercise 6, page 56)

Place your feet over a chair. Soften your lower back and relax
it onto the floor. Place your hands on your hip flexors and other
muscles at the front of your thighs; this will help you determine
whether you are able to relax them a little more (see page 56 for
further details).

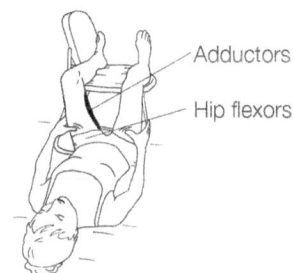

Hip flexor stretches (Exercise 49, page 133)

Go into a kneeling position with one leg forward. Place the right leg behind and
tuck the pelvis under until you can feel a stretch on the front of the right thigh.
Do not over-arch the back. Repeat on the left leg.

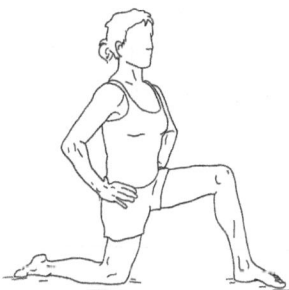

Lower-back releases (Exercise 32, page 117)

Lie on your back and hug both knees to your chest. Push the knees outwards
into your hands, but still keep your knees as close as possible to the chest. You
should feel a gentle stretch of your lower back.

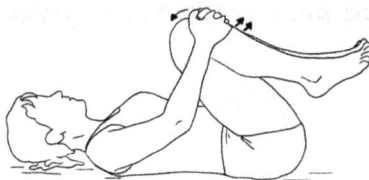

Hamstring stretch (Exercise 39, page 125)

Lie on your back and hug one knee up to the chest. Place your hands around the back of your thigh and keep the other knee bent. Gradually straighten and bend the raised knee to stretch the hamstrings. Pull the toes back towards you and this will also stretch the calf muscles. Repeat on each side.

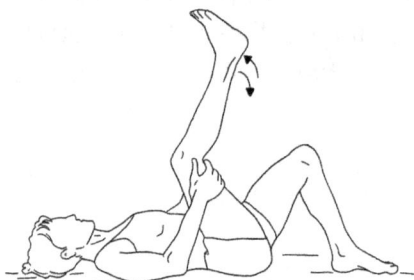

Four-point kneel (Exercise 34, page 118)

Go onto your hands and knees; keep the knees wider than your hips. Gently move your hips backwards, over and onto your legs. You should feel a stretch of your lower back and hips.

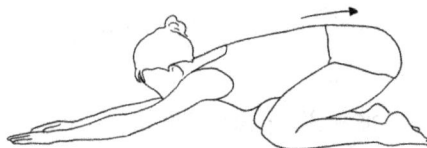

Four-point kneel for core stability (Exercise 14, page 97)

On your hands and knees, let your lower abdomen relax towards the ground. Do not let your back over-arch; keep it as relaxed as possible. Breathe in; as you breathe out, draw your pelvic-floor muscles and lower abdominals towards your spine. Maintain a gentle, submaximal contraction while you continue to breathe in and out comfortably four or five times. Be sure not to let your head drop downwards and keep your shoulder-blades drawn back and down.

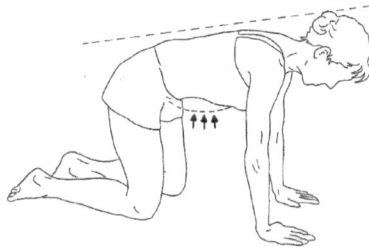

Stability exercises while supine (Exercise 9, page 94)

Place one hand on your upper chest and the other on your lower abdominals.

Inhale; as you exhale, engage your lower abdominals. Keep the lower back relaxed but maintain contact with the floor. Take four or five breaths while maintaining this gentle contraction.

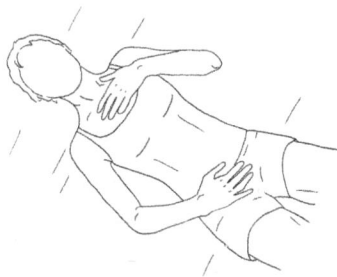

Extend arm and leg (Exercises 17 & 18, page 99)

To progress your lower-abdominals exercises, raise your arms at right-angles to the floor; keep the shoulders drawn back and down. Next, keep your lower abdominals engaged as you extend your leg a little way out and then bring it back in. Alternate, repeating four or five times with each leg. The goal is to keep your lower back in contact with the floor while you extend your right hand backwards and above your head, at the same time as extending your left leg. Repeat this on the other side; left hand above the head as you extend your right leg. Repeat four or five times on each side.

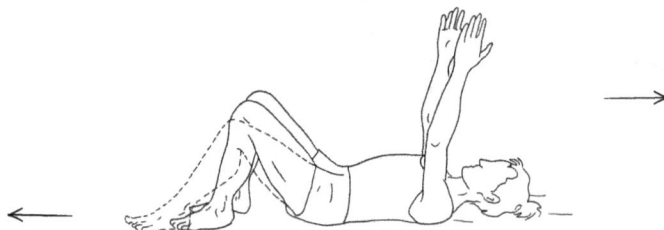

3. SWAY BACK

Defining features

The overall impression is that people of this postural type carry all of their weight too far forward over their hips. They are often over-flexible, or hypermobile (see page 122), and tend to stand with their knees locked into hyperextension. Also common is forward head and neck posture and stiffness of the thoracic spine.

Specifics

People with sway back can have some or all of these characteristics:

▶ hypermobility in all joints

▶ a tendency to stand with the knees and hips locked into hyperextension

▶ the appearance of strong, over-developed calf and quadriceps muscles, usually associated with weak gluteals

▶ hips that readily click due to over-lengthened hip flexors, or

▶ hypermobility only in the hips and shoulders, associated with stiffness of the thoracic spine.

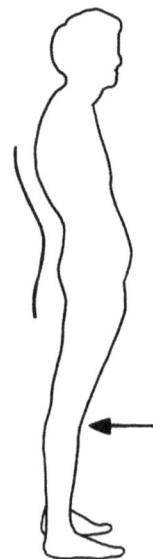

Postural tip

To counteract a sway back, think tall, soften the knees, shift your weight onto your heel bones, and engage the lower abdominals.

While standing, unlock your knees and shift your body weight a little backwards so that your hips are over your heels. Imagine a grape under the arch of the foot; lift your weight off the grape without clawing your toes. Lengthen the space across the front of the chest and draw your shoulders back and down. Try standing on a small wedge about five centimetres higher at the front. This can help you to find a more balanced centre of gravity and allow your core muscles to engage more automatically.

SUGGESTED EXERCISES FOR SWAY BACK

For sway back, focus on stability exercises, improve your balance, and pay attention to posture during the day. Tightness or soreness in your back after prolonged standing will usually be caused by your body's tiring and by giving in to your hypermobility. Do not overdo the stretches, especially if you are hypermobile. Your regime should give priority to strengthening the gluteals, lower abdominals and shoulders.

Hip flexion to extension (Exercise 29, page 109)

While standing, hug your knee; keep it at about 90 degrees to the body. Stand tall and maintain your balance. Once you can achieve this, extend the leg behind you. Repeat three to five times on each side.

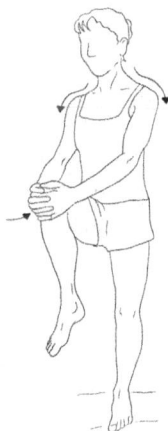

Stork (Exercise 30, page 109)

While standing, use your right hand to take hold of your right ankle and place it on the inside of your left thigh. The goal is to maintain this position for 30 to 60 seconds with perfect balance and ideal alignment of hips and arms. Repeat three or four times on each side.

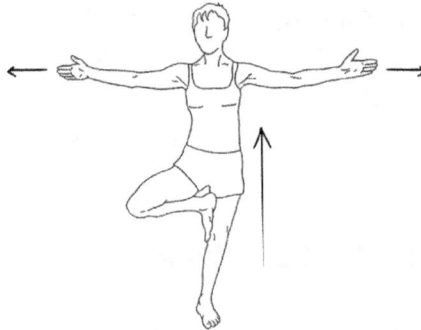

Walk on beam for stability (Exercise 73, page 237)

Stand on a soft beam or on a plank of wood. The goal is to keep the neck and shoulders relaxed, engage your core muscles then progress to moving one leg forward and back. Ideally, you should be able to maintain your balance easily. This exercise challenges all of your stability muscles and will help you achieve better overall posture.

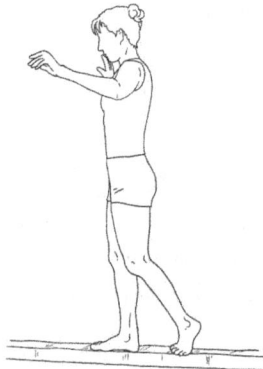

Side of spine stretch (Exercise 68, page 158)

Being highly flexible in your hips and shoulders (hypermobile) can often lead to stiffness in your mid back. This exercise can help you stretch this area of your back. While sitting, bend your left leg, loop a towel around your right foot and hold the ends in your left hand with your right hand placed on your left knee. Then look under your left arm and pull upwards into the side of your spine on the left side. Repeat on the right side.

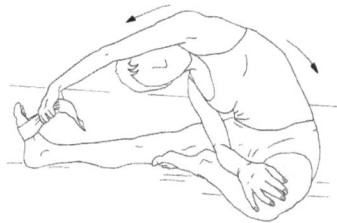

⚠ **CAUTION:** If you are not hypermobile, this exercise is not suitable for you.

Core stability while lying on a foam beam (Exercise 74, page 239)

All supine stability exercises can be made more fun and more challenging if you do them lying lengthways on a foam beam. Maintain a gentle activation of your core muscles as you extend one leg out and then draw it back in again. Repeat four or five times on each side. Progress to doing this exercise with your arms extended at 90 degrees to your body while you float one leg up and off the ground and then place it back down. Repeat on alternate sides. To challenge yourself even further, let one knee drop out to about 30 degrees to the side. Repeat on both sides of your body.

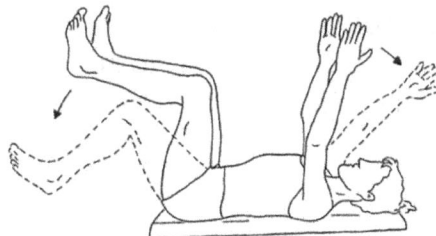

Prone stability (Exercise 22, page 102)

Lying face down, draw your shoulders back and down. Now engage the gluteal muscles on the right side of your body. Do not let the pelvis drop or tilt downwards as you flex your knee to 90 degrees. Repeat four or five times with each leg. The goal is to engage your gluteal muscles while your core muscles are still engaged.

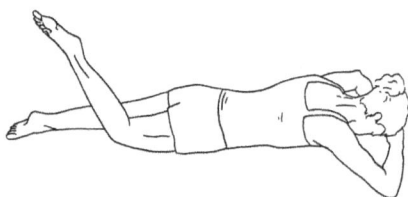

Strengthening gluteals by bridging (Exercise 26, page 107)

Lie on your back; imagine there is a line drawing your outside hip bones together, towards the mid-point. Lift your pelvis off the ground. Lower your body half-way down to the floor, then lift up again. Do not hyperextend the lower back. Repeat eight to ten times.

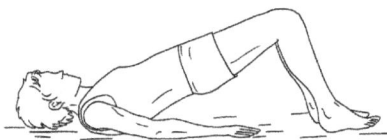

Mid-back stability using a band (Exercise 69, page 158)

While standing, take a piece of elasticised band in your hands. Draw the shoulders back and down and pull the band outwards, keeping the elbows at 90 degrees. The goal is to improve the stability and strength of the muscles of the mid back.

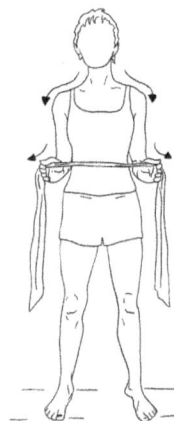

Advanced stability squat to hip extension (Exercise 31, page 110)

Balance on your right leg and place your left leg above your right knee. Keep the palms of your hands together as you extend the left leg behind you. This challenging exercise is excellent for improving your core muscles, overall stability and gluteal strength.

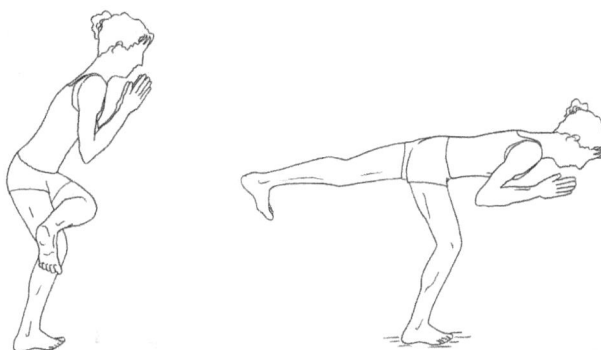

Strengthening gluteals (Exercise 89, page 251)

Take a cylindrical weight in your finger tips. As you go to sit in a chair, let the weight counter your downward movement by moving your arms slightly upwards and forwards. Stop before reaching the seat of the chair and reverse the movement. The goal is to use your gluteal muscles as you move upwards into a standing position again. Repeat six to eight times.

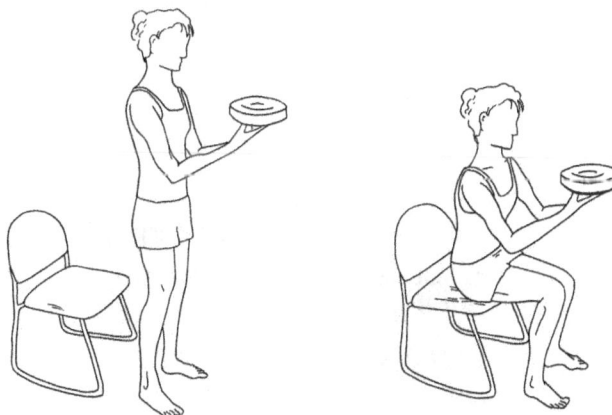

4. FLAT BACK

Defining feature

Some people have markedly reduced curves of the spine, or flat back. Instead of a natural inward arch or lordosis of the lower back, the overall impression is that the lumbar region looks unusually straight. The tendency is to compensate for this with a forward head and neck position. Those with a flat back tend to be stiff in the hips, hamstrings, calf muscles and often the shoulders. Being stiff in all of your joints is called hypomobility. The remedy is stretching and improving overall upper and lower body flexibility.

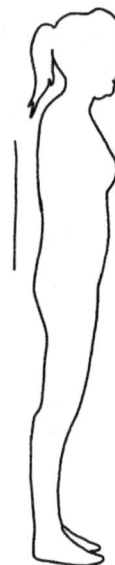

Specifics

Commonly associated with flat back are:

▶ posterior pelvic tilt

▶ stiffness and restriction in thoracic spine extension (arching backwards)

▶ weak gluteal muscles

▶ stiff hips, usually with limited internal rotation

▶ tight hamstrings and calf muscles, and

▶ forward head and neck posture.

Postural tip

When sitting or standing during the day, try increasing the inward arch of the mid and lower back. This will stop you feeling so stiff in the lower back and mid back when you need to stand or sit for a long time. This postural adjustment will also help correct a forward head and neck position.

SUGGESTED EXERCISES FOR FLAT BACK

Four-point kneel to increase lumbar lordosis (Exercise 34, page 118)

Go onto your hands and knees; keep your knees wider than your hips. As you stretch your pelvis back over your feet, try to keep a slight inward curve of your lower back.

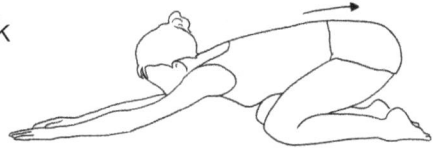

Mid-back stretch while lying on your side (Exercise 64, page 156)

Lie on your side, extend your arms out the front and place your palms together. Now extend one arm up, across your body and behind you. Follow your hand with your eyes; this will allow your head to move comfortably as you stretch your arm. You may need to rest your head on a rolled-up towel or pillow to do this exercise. The goal is to stretch your mid back and improve the flexibility of your shoulders.

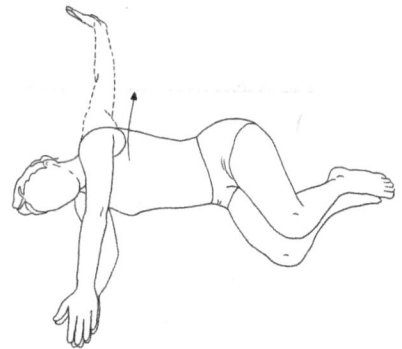

Mid-back stretch while standing; posture check (Exercise 51, page 143)

Stand with your back against a wall. Outwardly rotate the hands, keeping your elbows close to your side and at 90 degrees. The goal of this exercise is to improve your mid-back flexibility, especially into extension. Repeat the outward rotation of your arms two or three times. You can also do this easily while sitting in a chair.

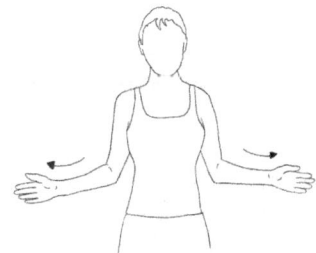

Stretching into the thoracic spine (Exercise 35, page 118)

While lying face down, place your hands under you, slightly wider than your shoulders. Stretch upwards and into your mid back. Do not over-extend into your lower back. Engage your lower abdominals; this will help you avoid over-arching and collapsing into your lower back. You should feel the stretch only in your shoulders and mid back.

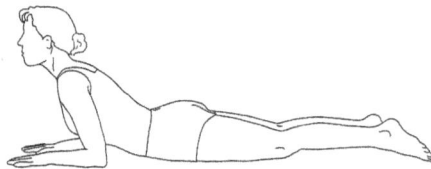

Hamstring stretches (Exercise 39, page 125)

Lie on your back and hug your right knee to the chest. Place your hands around the back of your right thigh; keep the left knee bent. Gradually straighten and bend the right knee to stretch the hamstrings. Pull the toes back towards you; this will stretch your calf muscles. Repeat on the other side, bringing the left knee to the chest.

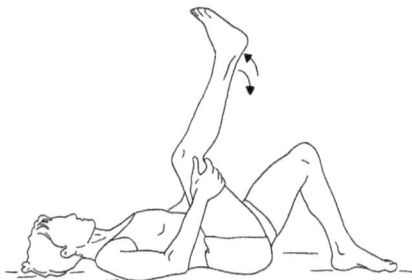

Hip flexibility stretches (Exercise 41, page 127)

Loop a towel around the left foot and hold the ends in your right hand. Draw the left leg across your body. Push into the left hip to increase the effectiveness of the stretch. Repeat with the right leg.

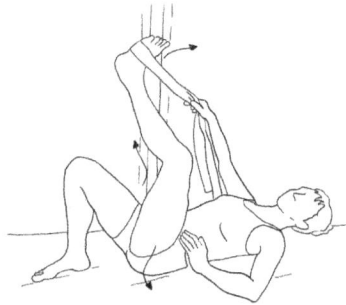

Gluteal strengthening (Exercise 26, page 107)

Lie on your back; imagine a line drawing your outside hip bones together, towards the mid-point. Lift your pelvis off the ground. Lower your body half-way to the floor, then lift up again. Do not hyperextend the lower back. Repeat eight to ten times.

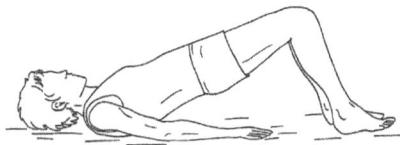

 Notes from the clinic

Do you have a lateral curve in your spine?

Most of the time, having a mild lateral curve in your spine poses no problem. It could be caused by a difference in the length of each leg. If so, you will need to find out whether the difference of leg length is causing back fatigue, which could also be caused by weak core and back muscles. The body can usually cope with a difference of up to five millimetres in the length of each leg without resulting pain.

The first postural aspect to consider is how you stand. If you have a shorter leg, you will tend to stand with the longer leg flexed and most of your weight on the shorter leg. If you are aware of doing this, try standing with your weight evenly balanced between both legs when possible, and do hip flexor stretches on the side of the longer leg (see Exercise 49, page 133).

If lower back pain persists after standing, try a heel raise inside your shoe on the side of your shorter leg (you need to do this regularly for at least three months). You will find out whether this heel raise is part of the solution to your back pain if you can stand more easily with your weight distributed evenly on both legs, and if your back no longer aches after long periods of standing.

In correcting a difference in the length of your legs, a long-term solution is to use an orthotic (a special shoe insert). It must measure only half the difference in leg length, to avert any strain in other areas of your body. If possible, consult a podiatrist, who will advise on whether you should use an orthotic with the heel raise incorporated, or whether the heel raise alone is the appropriate solution.

Postural habits you can change

When you start to change your postural habits, you will need to give yourself regular prompts; but after a while, new habits will become automatic.

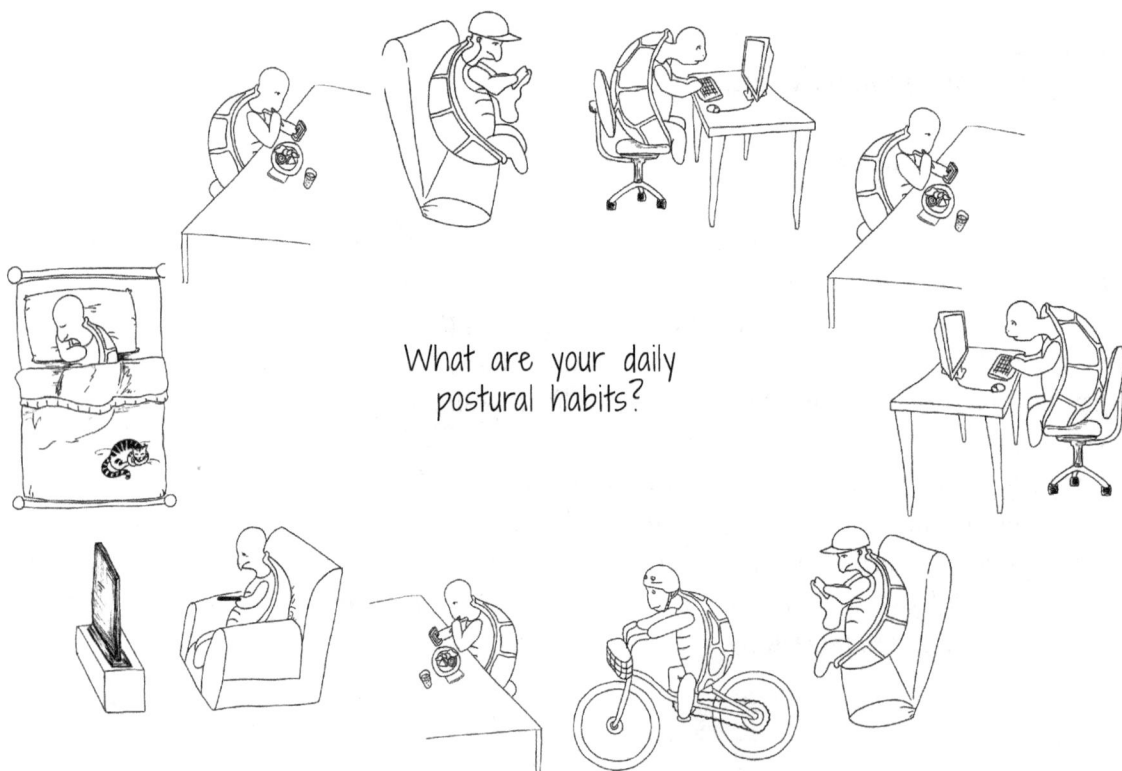

What are your daily postural habits?

You could sit, as many people do, from morning to night: on the way to work, in front of a computer, travelling home, relaxing at the end of the day and when using phones and other devices. After all that sitting, you curl up and sleep. Such consistent sedentary habits will make you feel old and stiff in the joints.

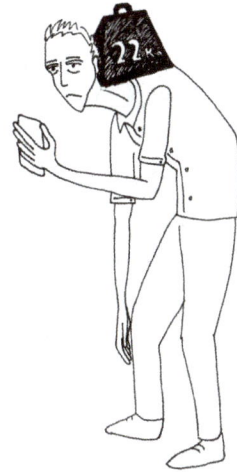

Research shows that regular users look at phones and other devices about every six minutes. The problem comes from leaning into the device and staying in a fixed flexed position for long periods.

If you have your head forward at an angle of greater than 45 degrees, this equates to putting from 22 to 27 kilograms of pressure onto the base of the neck.

Improving postural habits is a must. Here are some changes you can make immediately.

Sitting postures

When sitting at the desktop or using a laptop, these are strategies that will improve your posture and reduce the risk of back pain:

▸ Connect the laptop to a monitor and external keyboard when possible.

▸ Keep the mouse close to your body and keep elbows at about 90 degrees.

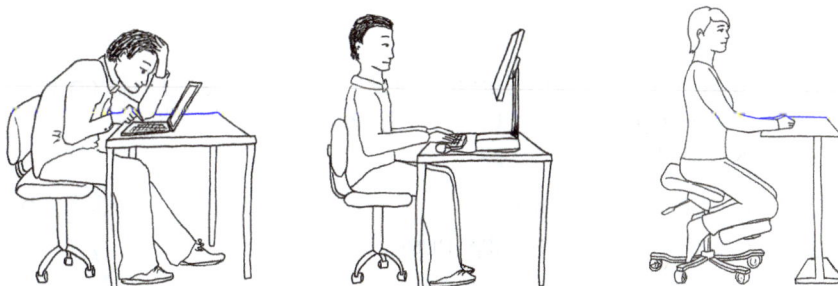

- ▶ Use a chair with a supportive back rest, or use a different style of chair such as a stool with knee rests.

- ▶ Take breaks from your regular chair and sit on a fitball for a while. Probably best to do this at home so there is no risk of injury through using this at work. Using the fitball gives your postural muscles a prompt to stay engaged.

- ▶ Keep your knees free so that you can rotate and move and not get stuck, for instance by having a filing cabinet next to you on one side.

- ▶ Place the monitor at eye level so that your eyes and head are not flexed forward.

- ▶ If you use reading glasses, have your eyes checked to see whether you need a prescription that includes an adjustment for different focal points. You will need this if your work involves looking at a document on the desk then at your computer screen.

- ▶ Use a document-holder next to your screen.

- ▶ If possible use voice activation for dictation, to shorten the time spent typing.

- ▶ On an uneven surface, use a foot stool or a small rolled-up towel under your feet. This will help you make small adjustments in your posture.

- ▶ Sit on a soft cushion so that the muscles in your spine are getting some small movements.

Additional tips

- ▶ Place a picture where you can see it, showing a calm and relaxing place, or a scene that makes you laugh, to keep your stress levels down.

- ▶ Look up and to the corners of the room in which you are working; this will prompt your eye and neck stability muscles.

- ▶ Prompt your core muscles by thinking about standing but do not stand; maintain this slightly taller posture.

▸ Push your body up a little through your hands; this will improve the inward curve of the spine and help align the upper body.

▸ Relax your neck and shoulder muscles before they begin to tighten.

▸ Place your hand on your shoulder at regular intervals to check whether your neck and shoulder muscles are relaxed (see Exercise 54).

▸ Do a small flutter with one hand, as if shaking water off. This prompts your postural muscles.

▸ Throw a small soft ball in the air; you need to keep adjusting your posture to achieve this.

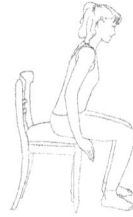

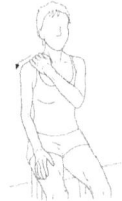

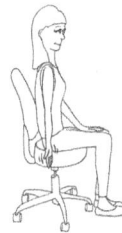

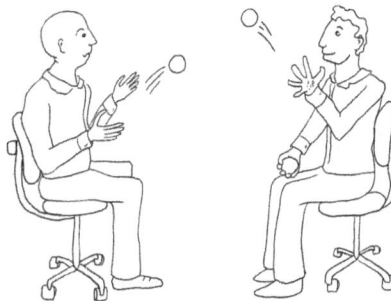

▸ Keep an elastic exercise band on your desk; do external rotations to loosen and activate the shoulder muscles.

▸ Drink water regularly. Your brain and your muscles need this to prevent tiring and slumping.

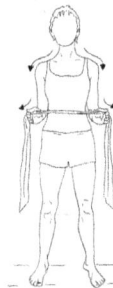

The use of a standing desk

Choosing to stand while you work depends on the type of work you do and is a personal preference.

Standing for some hours during the day has been shown to have many health benefits. However, if you are new to a standing desk, you might grow tired, lean on the desk and slump.

My recommendation is to alternate between sitting and standing. Alternatively, on top of your current desk, place an adjustable height stand that can be elevated.

When using a standing desk, place a support such as a book under one foot; this will take pressure off your lower back.

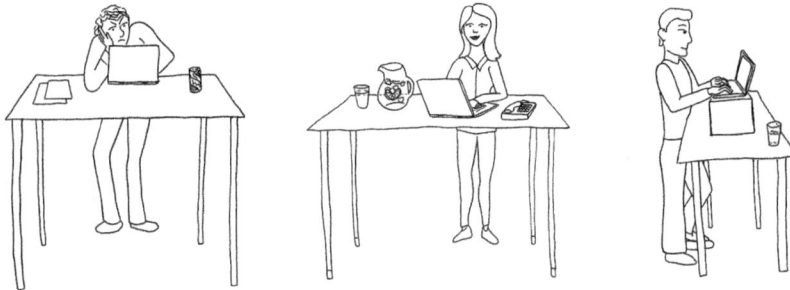

Take regular breaks

Here are some tips for back health while working at a desk:

▸ Get up and move every 60 minutes. Walk up and down the fire stairs, or use the stairs instead of the lift if possible.

▸ If circumstances allow, hold meetings outside while you go for a walk.

▸ Locate the printer at a distance from your desk.

▸ Try not to eat lunch at your desk. Maybe you could fit in a 30-minute exercise session and then eat your lunch.

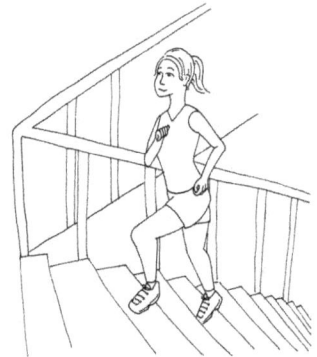

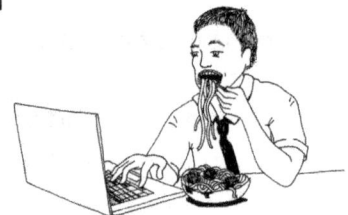

▸ When you take a break, seek a wall where you could throw a basketball. Organise a hoop if possible.

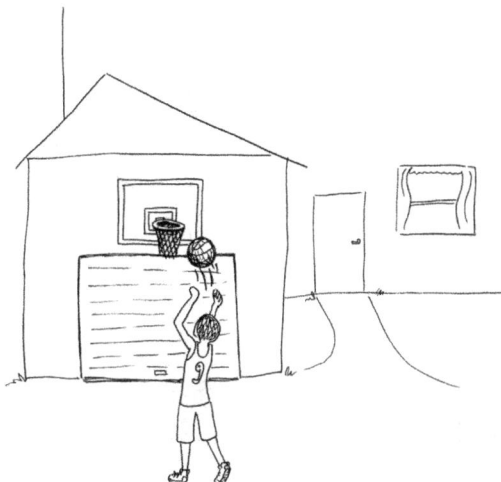

Use a pulley to keep the shoulders relaxed

If possible, attach a pulley securely to a wall and use it to loosen your neck and shoulders. This could also be hooked into a closed doorway. Be sure to put it on the side where there is no risk of the door being opened. Control the movement as you gently stretch each arm up and down. Keep the elbows bent; the distance you place the pulley away from the door will determine how much stretch you can achieve for your mid back.

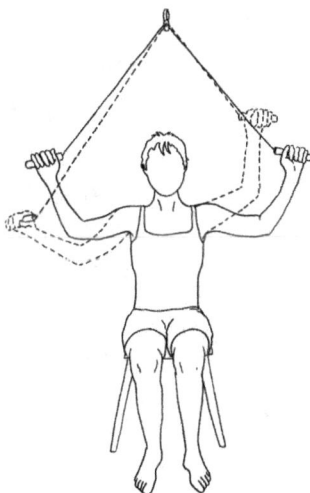

Imagine a piano with a keyboard under your feet and you are playing it with your toes. The amount of concentration required to do this gives your postural muscles a bit of a prompt. Be sure you glance away from the screen when you play the imaginary piano.

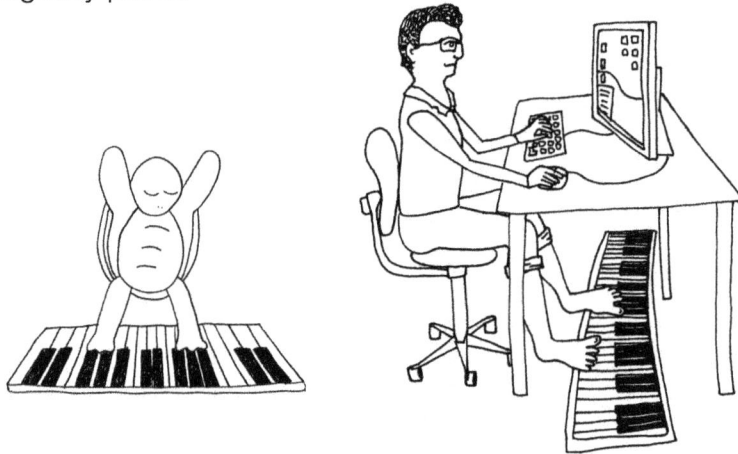

No matter how excellent your ergonomics are, you need regular breaks and routine adjustments to your posture; otherwise, postural fatigue and unnecessary aches and pains will set in.

 Notes from the clinic

What is good posture?

When I tell a client that their poor neck and shoulder posture is contributing to their back pain, they sit up straight into what they think of as "perfect" posture.

However, this is not good posture; it is too rigid. If you use the wrong muscles to correct your posture, a few minutes later you will collapse back to your stooped position. You know that you could not sit so rigidly all day.

Check your posture at unpredictable times.

Permit a colleague to take a photo of you while working at your desk or laptop when you least expect it. Your posture, captured in an unguarded moment, might surprise you.

Show a photo of your work station, from the sides, and the front, to your health professional. This will help to quickly identify the small ergonomic improvements that can be made, to take pressure off your neck or back.

When to use a postural brace

The various postural braces can be helpful as a reminder to adjust your posture. But you should use one for only about an hour, unless your health professional has advised you otherwise. If you know, for instance, that you tire in the afternoon, briefly use the brace then take it off again. The potential problem is that you can still tire with the brace on and your head and neck can still collapse forward. This will aggravate pain in your neck or mid back.

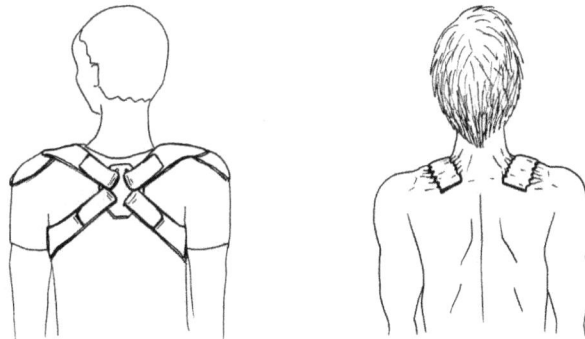

Just bunching your upper trapezius muscle with adhesive tape can be an easy and helpful alternative to a brace. You will need someone to put it on for you and you can keep it on for a full day.

Standing and walking

Think tall, but be at ease. Remember to relax the shoulders and breathe from the diaphragm.

Remember that postural sway and flutter can prompt your core muscles (refer to Chapter 5 for a reminder of how to use these cues to improve your posture).

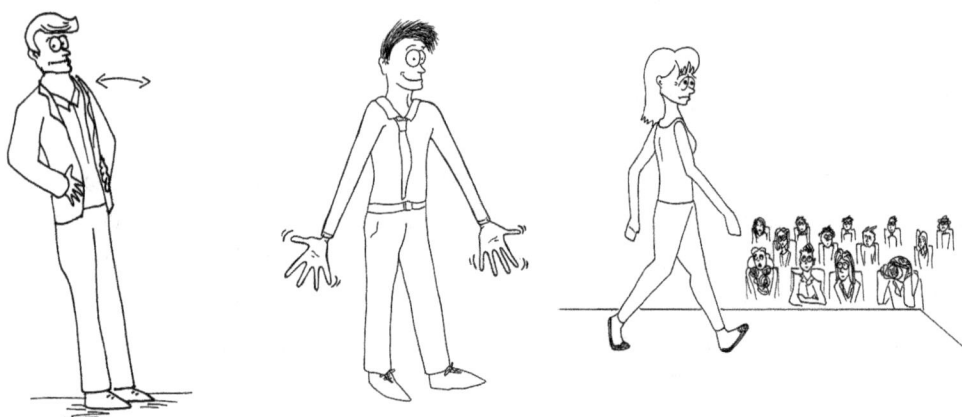

At the bus stop

Wherever you are, there is always some small movement you can do to adjust your posture. Poor posture and fatigue set in most readily when you stand in one position without moving.

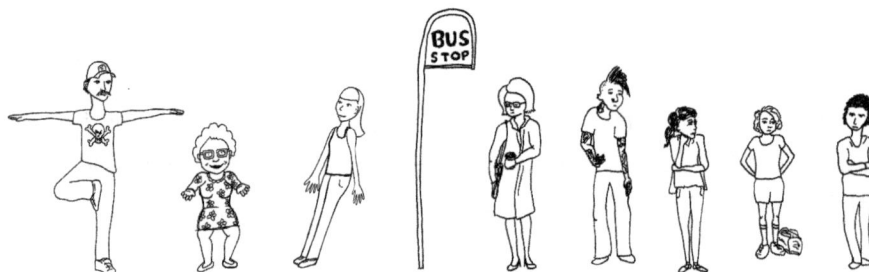

📖 *Notes from the clinic*

Are high heels bad for my back?

High heels increase the arch in your lower back and can cause excessive strain when standing for a long time. They can also tighten the hip flexors. Both can contribute to back pain.

Ways around the problem can include wearing jogging shoes to work and putting your heels on when you arrive, if your work requires you to wear them. If you have back pain, do not wear high heels. If you are seeking extra height, choose fashionable shoes that have a supportive arch and a platform right across the sole. Do not wear heels that are extremely high; you will risk sustaining other injuries such as an ankle sprain. As a guideline, heels higher than five centimetres have been shown to alter the curve of your lower back.

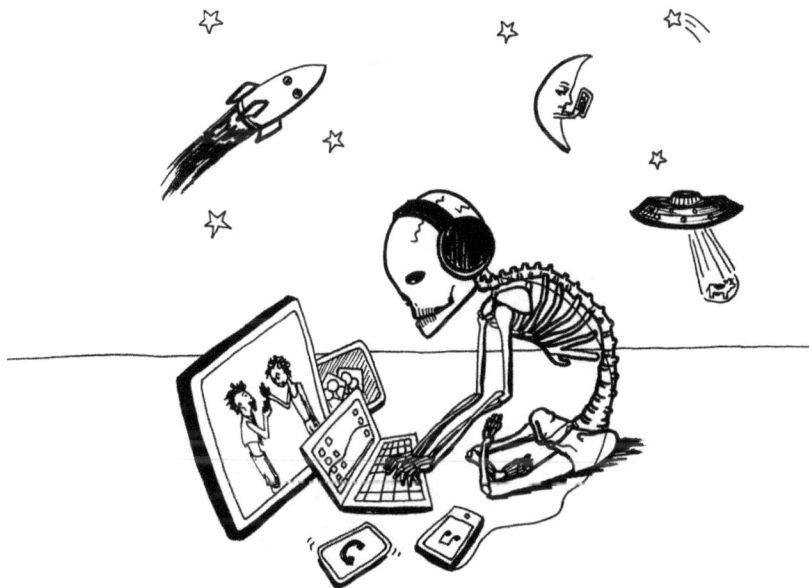

"I hope technology is not ageing me"

Mobile phone

Stand and try to use an earpiece when possible while speaking on your mobile phone. The goal is to try not to hook or hold the phone between shoulder and ear.

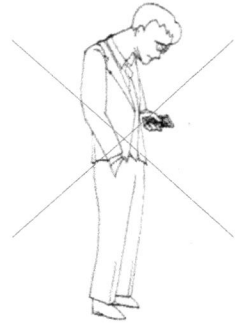

Stand on a dura disc (a rubber cushion filled with air) or a rolled-up towel. An unstable surface prompts your posture and core muscles.

Use both hands to text where possible.

If possible stand and push your foot backwards onto a wall. This will activate your postural muscles just a little.

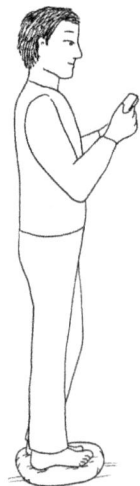

Tablet

Where possible rest your tablet against something, use both hands to type and use a keyboard when practical.

If at home, flex your knees up and rest the tablet on your legs.

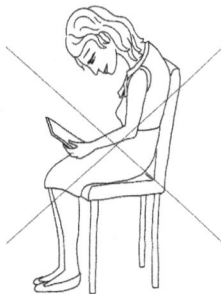

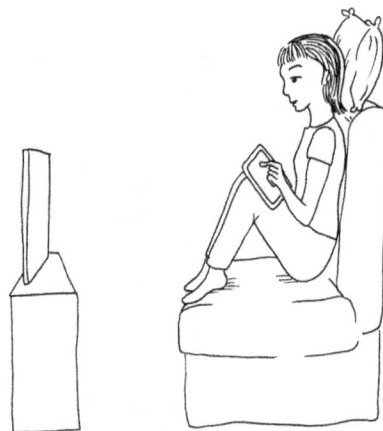

Watching TV

Have the TV in front of you so you are not looking to one side.

Resting with your feet up and knees slightly bent will relax the lower back; have your neck supported if possible.

If using a mobile device as well as watching TV, bend your knees up and rest the device on them as shown above, or place a small table across your knees.

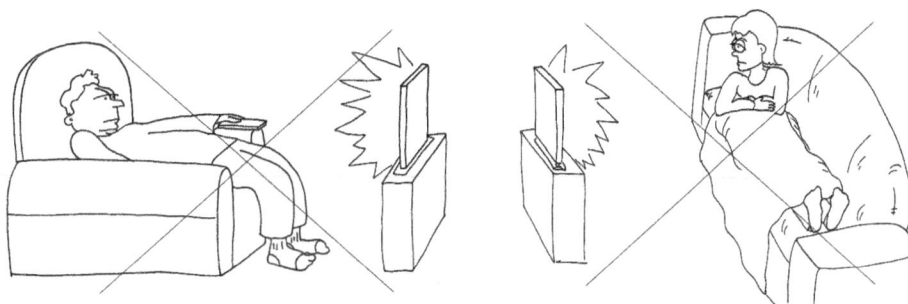

Driving

You might find that your back tightens after a long drive.

This is caused by not taking sufficiently regular breaks, and because in driving we use predominately our right leg in a continuously flexed position. This causes the right hip flexors to tighten.

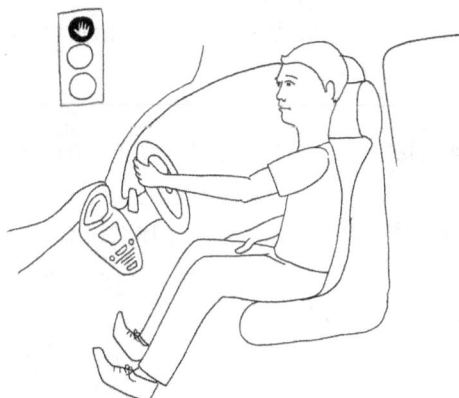

Try using a wedged cushion that is thicker at the back and thinner at the front, under your thighs. This will allow your hip flexors to relax a little more.

Another tip for driving: tighten and firm up your right quadriceps without moving your leg. Now relax the muscle and see if you can relax it more and more. You might need to place your hand on your thigh to check whether the muscle is totally relaxed. Do this exercise only when you are at the traffic lights or you will be too distracted. (Refer to Chapter 4 to check whether you are doing this hip flexor relaxation correctly.)

Truck drivers or other long distance drivers might also find that using a back support can be particularly helpful.

Sleeping

Lying on your side is the least stressful position for your back. Place a pillow between your knees and under your top elbow and this will keep your spine in a better alignment, with minimal rotation.

If you sleep on your back place a pillow under your knees.

Sleeping face down is stressful for your neck. Try placing a pillow between your knees and lying on your side. It will take time, but you should eventually be able to change your sleeping habit.

Just as your exact posture and flexibility are unique to you, so the mattress you prefer will vary. You might need a new mattress if the one you have sags and leaves an indent where your body lay through the night, or if your back is stiff and sore on waking in the morning. When you are purchasing a mattress, take the time to lie on different kinds before you make your final decision. A new mattress will improve your sleep; your neck and back should feel better in the morning.

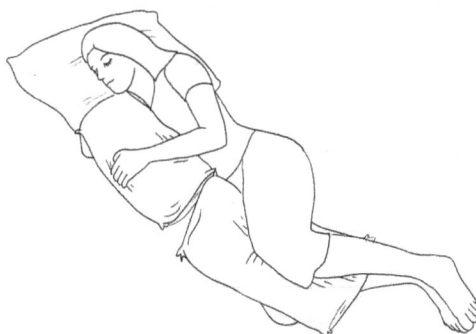

Reading a book before you sleep

Support your back by sitting up with pillows propped behind you. You might also need a pillow under your knees.

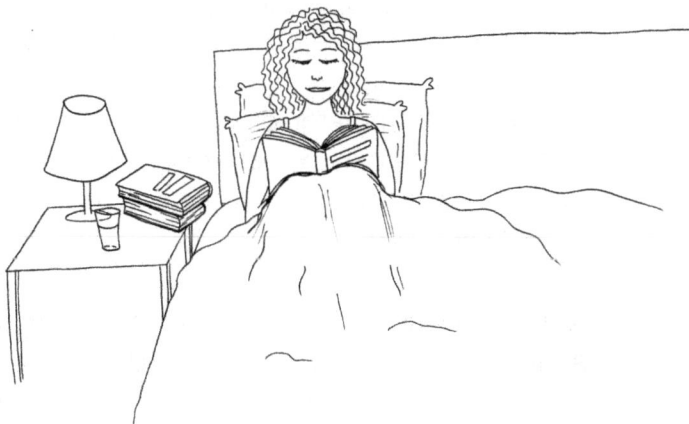

Parents need to know about teenagers' growing pains

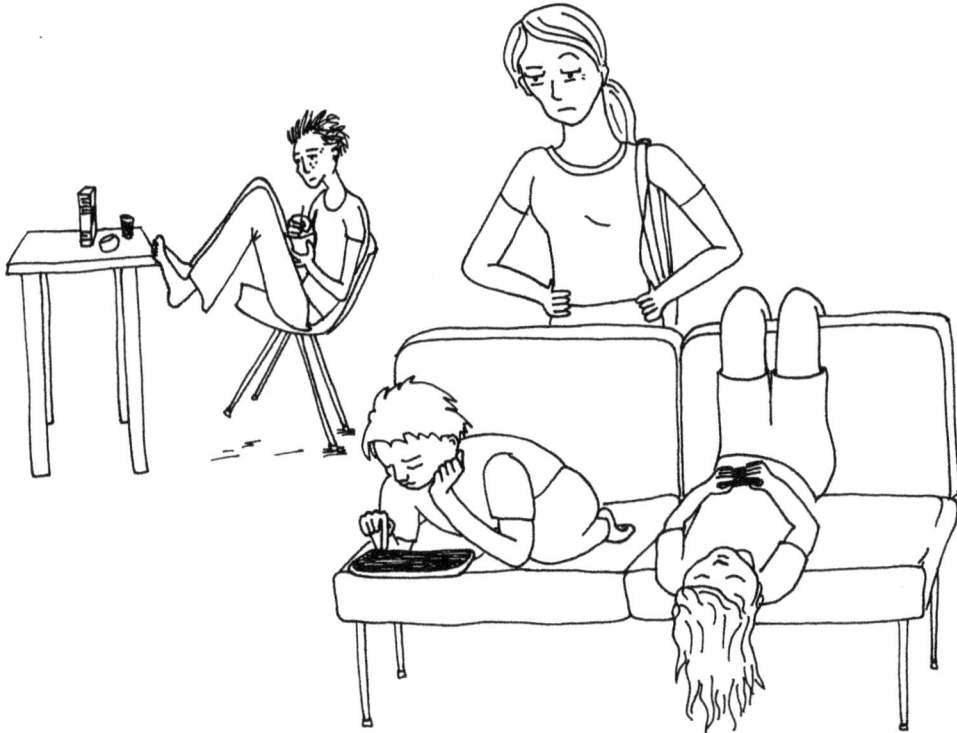

A teenager's growth spurt is the most critical time for parents to pay attention to their boy's or girl's posture and overall fitness. A boy's growth spurt usually occurs at 15 or 16 years of age; for girls, sudden growth happens earlier, at 10 to 12 years. Often, children can have more than one growth surge.

Growing pains are real. Bones grow more quickly than muscles, tendons and the sheath of nerves. This imbalance can explain some unpredictable teenage aches and pains. As a remedy for growing pains, the neural stretches outlined in Chapter 4 can often be highly beneficial.

Let your teenager know that the last bone in the body to mature is the collarbone. This means that their posture and upper body strength in the growing years influence their posture for the rest of their life. My teenage patients with neck or back pain sit up and listen when I tell them this.

Improving teenagers' posture and fitness

Excessive use of mobile phones and other electronic devices in a sustained forward head and neck position is creating the potential for the much too early onset of neck and back pain.

Below are tips to help teenagers cope with the changes that they are going through.

▸ Fitness is essential in the growing years. Teenagers must exercise at least three times a week; they should choose the type of exercise they enjoy or they will not stay committed to it. The exercise they prefer might change through their growing years.

▸ Scale back competitive ball sports and running when your child is going through a growth spurt. This will reduce the risk of tendon problems, particularly of the knee. The child might become disillusioned and cease all sport if they are injured.

▸ If possible, acquire a supportive chair and desk for the teenager.

▸ Provide a back pack that has a strap around the pelvis and place the heaviest items closest to the body inside of the pack.

▸ If possible convince your child to wear the pack at the front – not easy as this is not fashionable.

Get your teenager to try some of the following fitness, upper body strengthening and fun stability and co-ordination exercises. This will reduce the time they spend in a static posture. You should perhaps do some of these yourself first, particularly the co-ordination ones, before you ask your child to do them.

Set up a basketball hoop to encourage them to take a break.

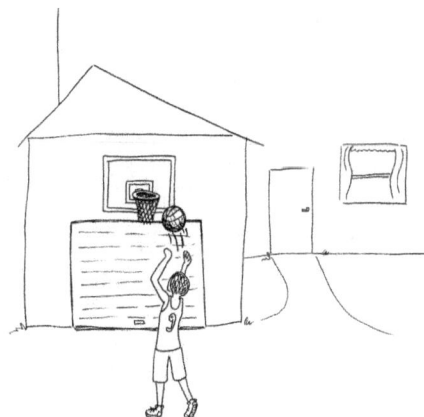

Check whether they can support their body weight through their arms. They should be able to.

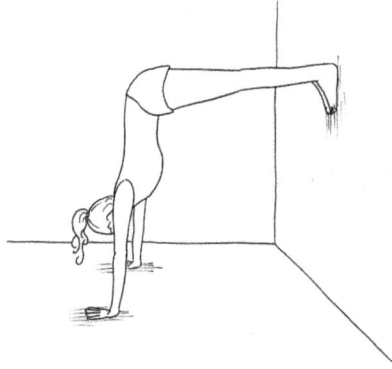

Excellent posture exercises

If your child is not strong enough to do a handstand, suggest that they keep a band on their desk, wrap it around their back and secure it between their thumbs. Four or five controlled movements, out to the front and back again, is an excellent mid back and neck strengthening exercise. Do this yourself first before you teach your teenager (see Exercise 70).

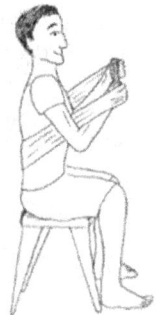

As well, check whether your teenager can balance on a foam beam while they throw and catch a ball.

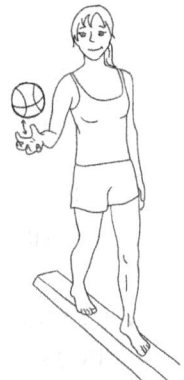

Try these co-ordination exercises

These are excellent ways to activate and train the brain as well as providing a break in study time.

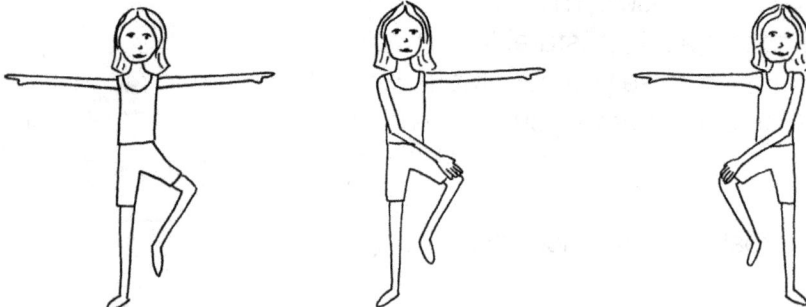

Stand with arms outstretched and tap one hand on the inside of the opposite knee. Do this exercise in front of a mirror to be sure that the knee does not cross over the midline of the body; that is, be aware of alignment.

Let the opposite arm and leg float out to the side.

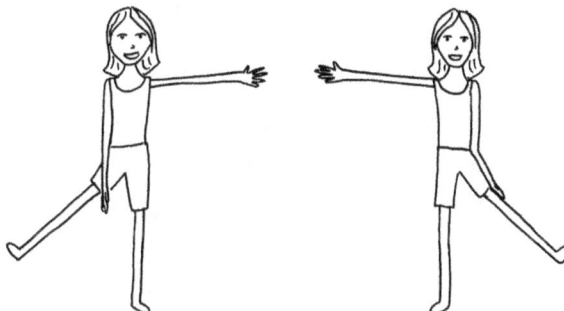

Bend the knees and put each hand on the same knee. Now tap your right hand onto your nose and your left hand onto the right ear. Swap hands and do it the opposite way.

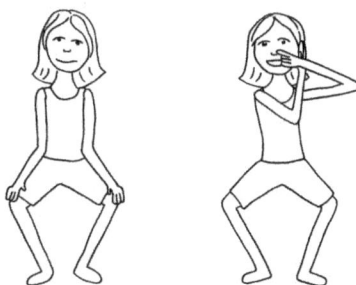

Your child of any age will have fun with these.

For younger children

A way to encourage good posture is to attach a child's iPad or other device to the fridge. Then your child will need to stand up straight to use the device, instead of slumping. This is a great tip for teachers too, who can attach pupils' devices to a classroom wall.

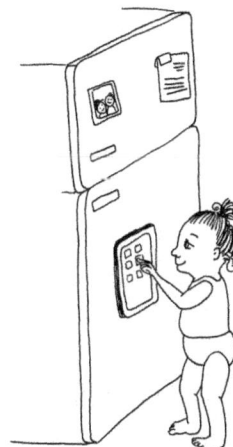

💡 Points to remember

▸ Use technology to help you not to age you.

▸ A combination of genetics and daily habits influence posture.

▸ Knowing your postural type will help you to know where to stretch and what to strengthen.

▸ Have someone take a photo of you in profile, when you are totally relaxed and not concentrating on trying to correct your posture. This will help you to identify aspects of posture that you need to improve.

〝☰ Actions to take

Take steps to improve your posture while sitting, moving around, standing, or lying down.

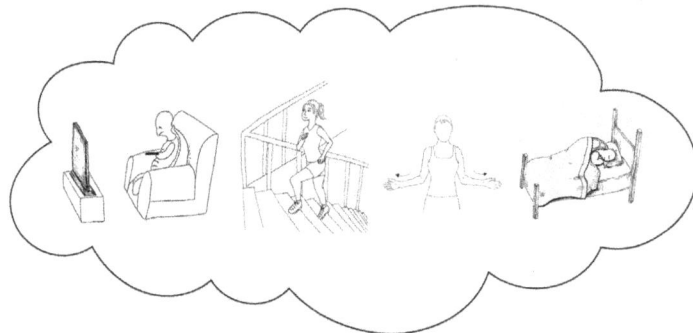

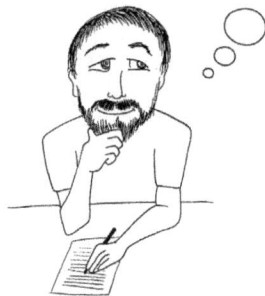

"I feel better just thinking about all the ways I can improve my posture. I definitely must consider trying them"

✎ **Notes**

10 Common diagnostic terms

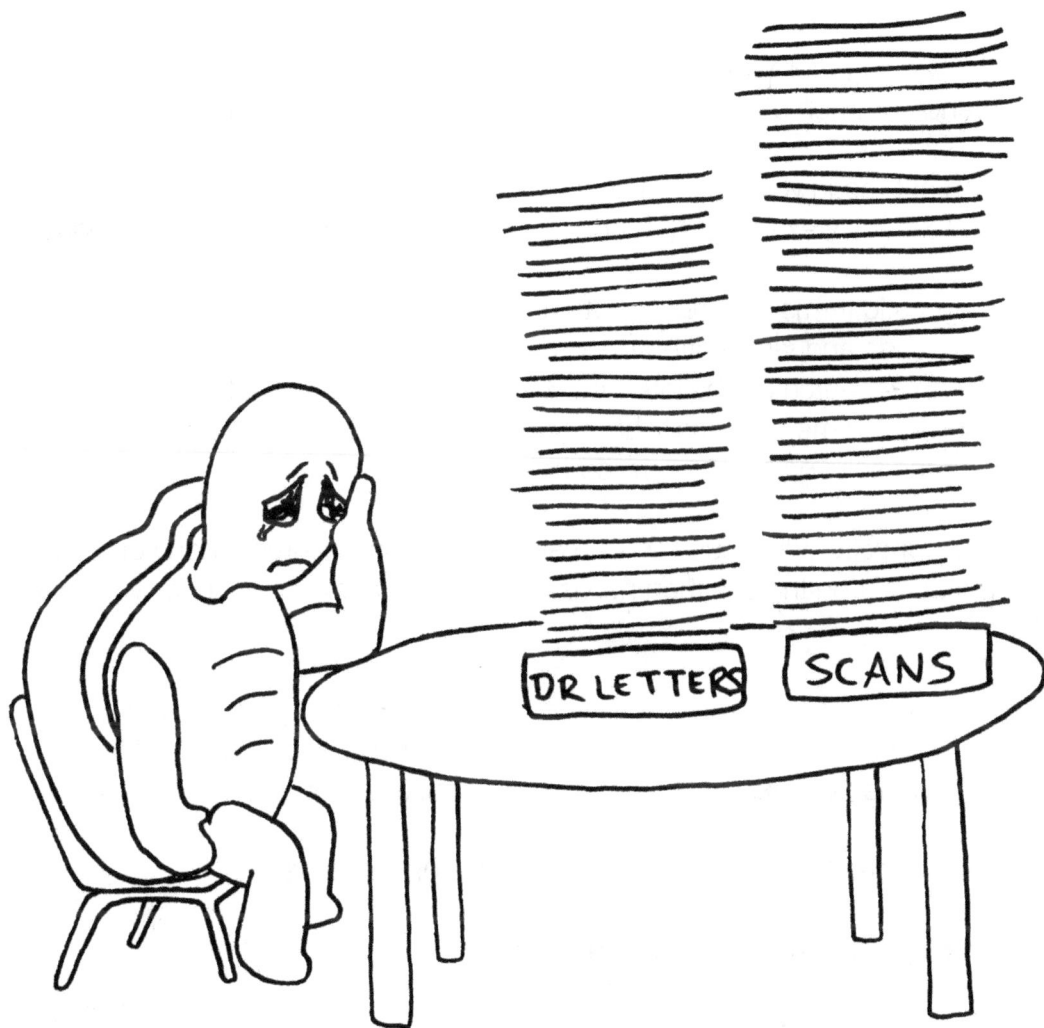

Understanding the language of back pain

Combining the information from radiological scans with your health professional's clinical findings is the best way to overcome back pain.

Before proposing more advanced and challenging exercises, you should understand common diagnostic terms that you may have heard over the years.

This does not mean you will be able to diagnose yourself, but the information will help you to identify exercises that should be omitted from your current program.

Most diagnostic terms describe what can be seen on a radiological scan. Well-meaning friends and family often become self-appointed experts in what these terms mean. A search on the internet, which most of my patients have done before consulting me, can easily have you thinking that your pain is far more serious or the solution much more complex than it is.

Often the opposite will occur. You can almost be disappointed when your scan is clear, because then there is then no visible anatomical explanation for your back pain.

The additional information from a scan enables your health professional to determine how this correlates with your description of your pain and to recommend the best exercises and strategies for your condition.

Below are some of the typical terms that you might have heard.

Slipped disc, disc bulge or protrusion

You may have heard a disc problem referred to as a slipped disc.

The disc does not and cannot slip out of place, but the outer layer of the disc can be strained. This shows as a bulge on a radiological scan and can be a normal, age-related finding. The degree of disc strain will determine whether it is classified as a disc bulge or a protrusion.

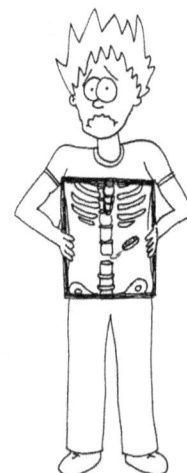

"Where has my disc gone?"

Research shows that a disc bulge might or might not be associated with pain. Anatomical changes on your scan are only part of the picture. Some patients bring a scan in to me with a disc bulge and have no pain; others are experiencing a lot of pain with no disc bulge.

With the appropriate clinical assessment, a disc bulge and the associated pain can be resolved by the exercises in this book.

If your pain is greater than eight out of ten (ten is extreme pain) and your pain is not settling with conservative treatment by your health professional, with exercise or with pain medication, I highly recommend that you consult a sports physician, orthopaedic or neurosurgeon. This is crucial if you have conditions that are not resolving, such as pins and needles in your leg, referred pain, constant night pain, or muscle weakness in the foot.

Surgery could be required to resolve your pain. It might be needed if the disc is creating persistent nerve pain. If surgery is required, the results should be more positive when you are as fit as possible and have good awareness and knowledge of your stability muscles.

Helpful tip

Below is an outline of postures that can aggravate your pain.

The lumbar disc more commonly bulges posteriorly (towards the back). This is usually because you have been in a sedentary or sustained flexed posture for a long time, then move too quickly or lift something too heavy.

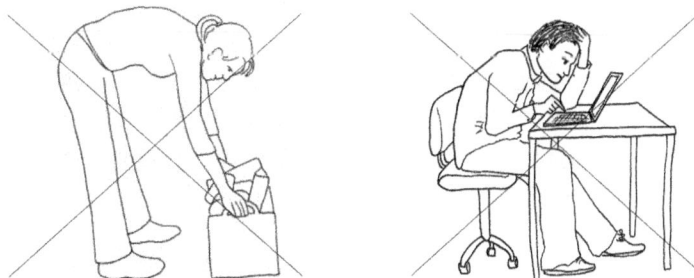

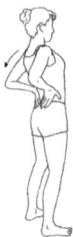

The solution is to take regular breaks; and reverse the flexed position your back is being used in, that is, stretch into extension.

Figure 23. An MRI (Magnetic Resonance Imaging) showing a mild disc bulge and disc degeneration. Either of these could be the cause of your back pain, but might not be

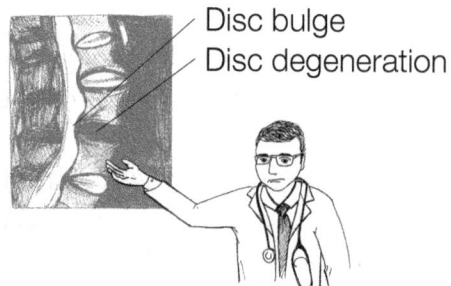

Disc degeneration

Disc degeneration does not mean that you need to stop exercising. It is a not a diagnosis by itself, nor a disease. With age (or excessive sport) fluid in the gelatinous disc between each vertebra reduces slightly; this will show as a darker area on an MRI. Disc degeneration is usually associated with reduced distance between each vertebra, which is a normal part of ageing. You might have noticed that you have lost a small amount of height as you have aged, or that you have become slightly stooped.

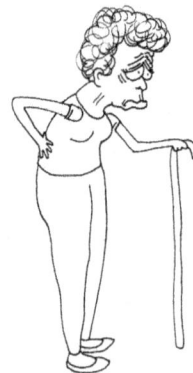

The bottom two vertebral levels in the lumbar spine (L4/L5 and L5/S1) and base of the neck (C5/C6) are the levels of the spine that take most of our postural overload. Sometimes there are bony spurs called osteophytes at the level of degeneration as well. The combination of these findings on scans is often termed spondylosis.

Such scan findings might contribute to some of your pain, but more often it is lower back stiffness or tightness in the neck muscles that you will be feeling. If your scans look like these conditions, it is vital to keep moving and find activities that do not feel painful. Your focus needs to be on the stretches covered in the chapters above for the neck and the back, more than on stability.

Research shows that the right nutrition can play a significant role in reducing some of the muscle stiffness associated with disc degeneration, so I would recommend that you consult a nutritionist to review your diet.

Not recommended: Unsupported back extension could cause or aggravate pain in the facet joints of your lower back.

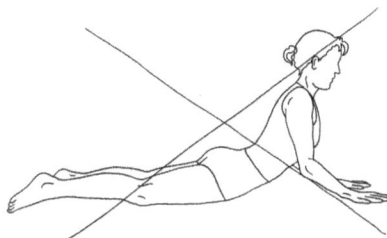

Recommended: You must still maintain extension of your spine. A less stressful way to achieve this is to lie on your side with your knees bent up, clasp your hands behind your neck and gently move your elbows away from each other (see Exercise 4).

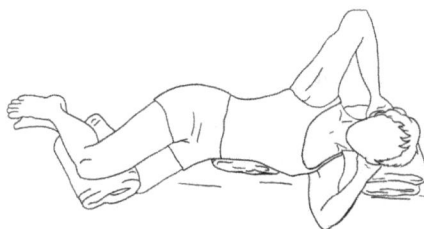

You could also try a gentle flexion stretch, hugging both knees to your chest each morning to start the day (see Exercise 33).

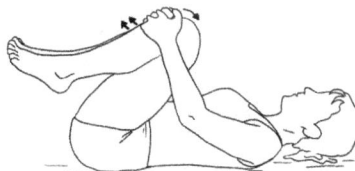

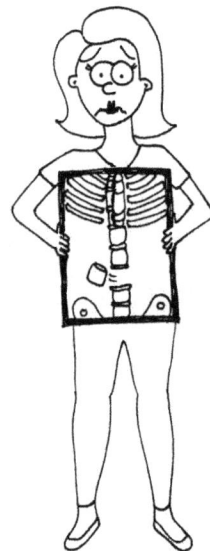 *Notes from the clinic*

Chronic pain is not a diagnosis

Many patients who consult me about longstanding pain explain that they have been told their diagnosis is "chronic pain". As health professionals, we sometimes use this term when a client has had episodes of pain for more than three months.

However, the most important thing to do in such circumstances is to find out why your brain is continually sending messages that it needs to protect your body. You might not be aware that you are doing this.

The focus of your treatment for recurring, longstanding pain would be to assess your radiological scans and consider whether the findings correlate with your current pain. Your treatment will then include the correct exercises for you and allow a review of your current thought patterns.

Slipped vertebra

On an X-ray film, a vertebra may appear to be misaligned with the others in your spine, for example by having slipped a few millimetres forward. Less frequently, a vertebra may slip backwards a little. The medical name for the forward slip is a spondylolisthesis; the backwards slip is called retrolisthesis.

In most instances, exercise can prevent recurrent instability or back locking that might be associated with this condition. Surgery is not usually required; when it is, the higher your overall fitness, and the stronger your stability muscles, the better the post-surgical results.

"I wonder where the vertebra that has slipped will show up..."

Helpful tip

Not recommended: Do not do extension exercises if you have a spondylolisthesis or retrolisthesis; such exercises will usually aggravate back pain.

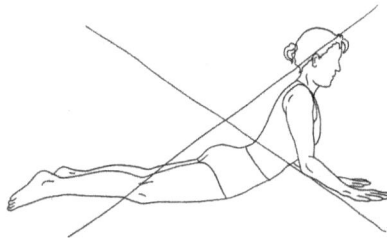

Recommended: Work with your health professional to learn the exercises that are most suitable for your condition. Each of the slipped verterba conditions requires a slightly different approach to exercise management.

Sciatica

When a disc bulges or protrudes it can press on one of the spinal nerves. Pressure on a nerve can also result from narrowing of the disc spaces in association with osteophytes. The nerve and its sheath can become inflamed. This can cause localised pain in the back or pain referred down into the buttock or leg. The latter is called sciatica. Anti-inflammatory medication might help ease sciatic pain. If some adhesions or catch points of the nerve sheath remain, you might feel this as tightness in your gluteal, hip or hamstring muscles.

The sciatic nerve runs adjacent to and sometimes through a deep muscle in the buttocks called the piriformis. Tightness in the piriformis could cause some sciatic-related pain.

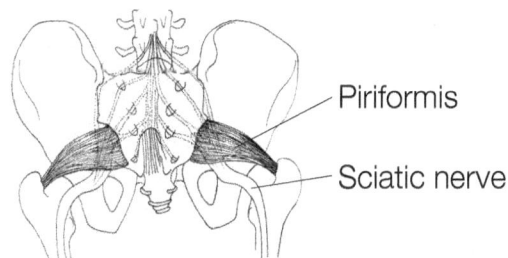

Piriformis

Sciatic nerve

Figure 24. Shows the sciatic nerve as it traverses deeply through the buttock and the back of the hip. It is closely related to the deep muscle called piriformis

Doing neural glides and outer hip stretches might relieve any tightness in the gluteals or sciatic pain. However, do not continue with this exercise if it increases your referred pain.

⚠️ **CAUTION:** I do not recommend neural exercises for a sudden, sharp episode of sciatic pain. In this instance, you should consult your health professional, who can advise on the appropriate strategies for pain relief.

Exercises to ease sciatic pain

These exercises are for chronic sciatic pain.

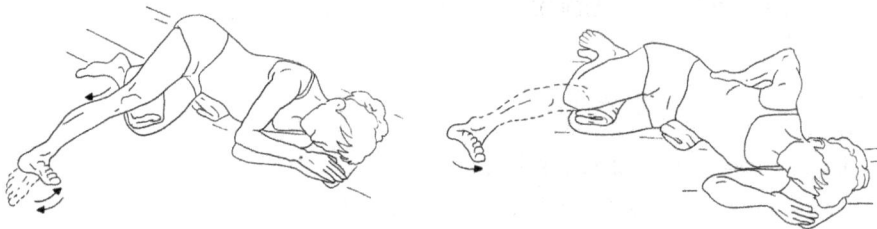

Do upper limb neural exercises first (see Exercise 3) and then those for the lower limb (see Exercise 4). If this does not aggravate your gluteal or leg pain, add the following outer hip stretch (see Exercise 41).

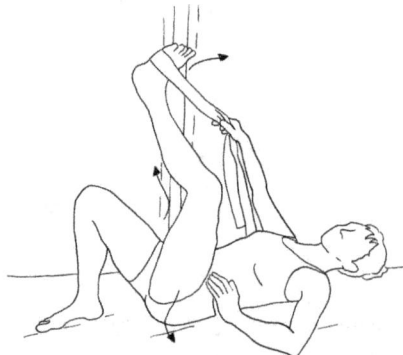

📖 *Notes from the clinic*

Injections are sometimes necessary for back pain

A guided injection while undergoing a CT scan might relieve pain. It could enable you to move more freely, regain confidence and start exercising again. It will also help to clarify your diagnosis.

Remember that pain is inhibiting the muscles from being pre-set and automatically supporting your back. The use of cortisone in pain reduction can enable you to move forward, but be realistic about your expectations. Do not rely on the injection alone to solve your pain. You will also need to address muscle weakness and tightness as well as paying attention to the way you think about pain.

Pelvic girdle pain: sacroiliac joint

Any pain affecting the joints, tendons, nerves or muscles of the pelvis is called pelvic girdle pain. The most common joint that can be problematic in this area is the sacroiliac joint. This is where the ilium (hip bone) joins the sacrum. You may experience this as pain slightly lateral and away from the midline of the spine. Sacroiliac joint pain is most commonly due to instability of the ligaments in this joint. While this can be caused by injury or other trauma, laxity in this joint is most commonly associated with pregnancy.

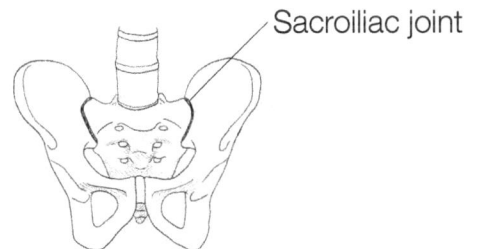

Sacroiliac joint

Research has shown that improving the strength of pelvic floor muscles, and strengthening all of the other core muscles, significantly reduces sacroiliac joint pain.

Find out whether you have stiffness in this joint, or laxity. Your health professional can assess and help you to determine what is happening. If you have laxity in the joint, the stability exercises for the core and gluteals outlined in previous chapters would be ideal.

 Notes from the clinic

Using a sacroiliac joint belt

Sacroiliac joint pain is common with pregnancy because of associated laxity of the ligaments. You might need to use a belt that is specifically designed to assist with stabilising this joint (ask your health professional about acquiring one). The belt should feel supportive and should reduce your pain. You should be able to do most of your core stability exercises without using the belt, provided that you have no pain. However, I would recommend using the belt during the day when you are more active and perhaps lifting and moving unpredictably. The goal is to wean yourself off using the belt as you get stronger.

Arthritis

A diagnosis of osteoarthritis does not mean that you should resign yourself to permanent back pain. Radiological findings showing that you have osteophytes or visible arthritis on many levels of your spine can be disconcerting. However, the best thing you can do is keep moving, do regular, gentle stretching and other exercises that do not worsen your pain. If you cannot walk far, try using a stationary bike or exercising in a pool. I have outlined some exercises in the next chapter to make this more fun and more interesting for you.

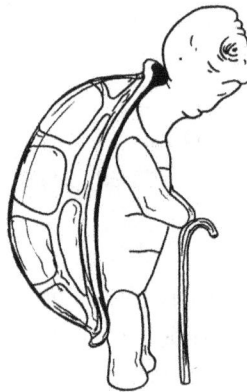

"I guess I should stop exercising?"

Discuss with your GP what medication would be appropriate for you. This is particularly important if you have been diagnosed with rheumatoid arthritis rather than osteoarthritis.

Helpful tip

Remember that better muscle function means less pain and more mobility. I recommend to patients who bring in scans with arthritic changes to consult a nutritionist or dietician. Low-grade inflammation in the body such as arthritis has been shown to improve with changes in one's diet.

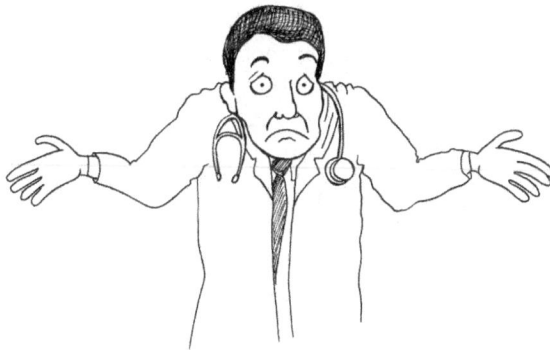

"Your diagnosis is non-specific low back pain"

Non-specific pain

Non-specific low back pain can be a helpful diagnosis. Sometimes you might hear it called idiopathic pain (no known cause).

This news can be frustrating but ultimately positive. It usually means that your radiological scans are clear. There is no anatomical structure on your scans which could explain why you have pain, and you might have had no specific incident or injury. This means that the proactive approach proposed in this book is perfect for you to put into action.

 Notes from the clinic

Your back is not "out"

Many of my patients tell me that their back or pelvis feels "out" although their scan is clear.

"I look in the mirror and can see I am standing twisted – I must need someone to help straighten me up – doubt I can fix this myself…"

On your radiological tests you will not see any vertebra out of place, even though you feel as if something is "out" and you often look twisted in the mirror.

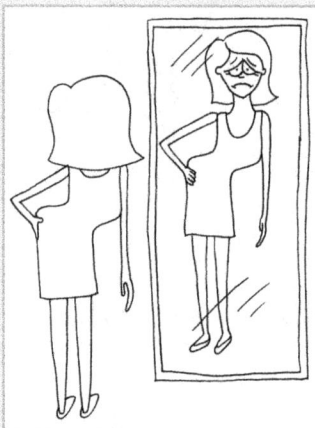

Your locked back is usually due to muscle spasm protecting an underlying muscle weakness, often from a previous episode of back pain. This weakness might cause the spine to lock at one vertebral segment. Think of your spine as a bike chain with one link locked, which stops the chain from moving and turning the bike wheel.

As outlined in earlier chapters, the muscles that usually compensate are the erector spinae in the back and the hip flexors and adductors, which usually tighten on one side more than the other. Test this by doing a hip flexor stretch and comparing the sides. Stretch more on the tight side; the back muscles will usually start to relax and you should look a little straighter in the mirror.

Start your stability and neural exercises as soon as possible. In combination with massage and mobilisation, an acute episode of back pain can usually be resolved in these ways. Your challenge however, is to troubleshoot. Why did your back lock? What activity might have caused it? What habits do you need to change to avert recurrent episodes of your back locking?

Once the pain resolves it is easy to neglect the basics. The goal is to maintain your overall fitness and keep doing stability and neural exercises, even when you are not in pain.

💡 ***Helpful tip:*** *In an acute episode of locking, you might need to wear a supportive back corset for a few days until the muscle spasm eases. As soon as possible, reduce use of the corset to occasions on which you are doing heavy or unexpected lifting, as required if you have young children.*

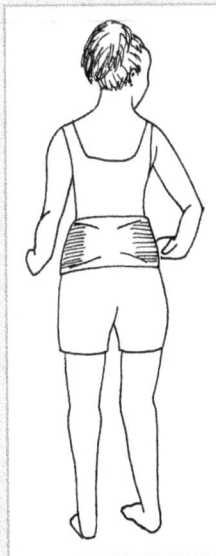

⚠ ***Caution:*** *If you are experiencing constant pain at night, pins and needles or numbness in your feet that is not settling with exercise or treatment, irrespective of your scan report, I would recommend you get a second opinion from another medical practitioner.*

Pain in the brain

Pain is experienced in the brain but maybe not in the way you think.

Traditionally, pain was explained this way: pain receptors throughout the body are activated when we are injured, sending a message to the brain; then a reaction occurs in the body. In an acute injury this does happen. The brain activates many responses to permit local healing of an injured area.

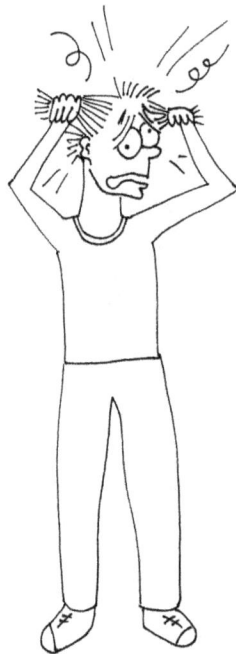

"They say my pain is in my brain - but I'm sure I'm not imagining it. I know I can feel pain - I know it's real. Why won't anyone believe me?"

However, advances in technology, including Functional Magnetic Resonance Imaging, have shown that areas of the brain associated with pain often stay reactive even though a local injury has healed. We learned in Chapter 3 that these changes in the brain are called neurotags. But sometimes the areas associated with pain in the brain do not correspond to the level or severity of an injury.

Consider examples of this phenomenon.

You can feel acute pain from a minimal injury such as stubbing your toe or a paper cut. Here is the sequence:

Pain sensors in the nerves in your toe or finger are activated.

The brain determines the appropriate response.

Pain centres in the brain are activated so that your body responds.

You pull your foot away, but soon you have forgotten about it and a few minutes later you are moving or walking normally again.

Pain centres in the brain calm down.

Alternatively, athletes and others can at times feel no pain, even though they competed with a major injury such as a broken bone.

When questioned at a later time, they often have no recollection of being in pain.

Often they only feel the pain after the adrenalin rush of the competition has passed.

There is a need to explain this discrepancy. The current explanation of pain, which you learned in earlier chapters of this book, is that pain is an output from the brain, a reaction to what all of your senses are telling you. The brain continually filters all the information it receives, then determines the appropriate response.

For instance, your body does not let you stub your toe again immediately after the first time you stubbed it. The message comes from the brain to protect you from hurting yourself again.

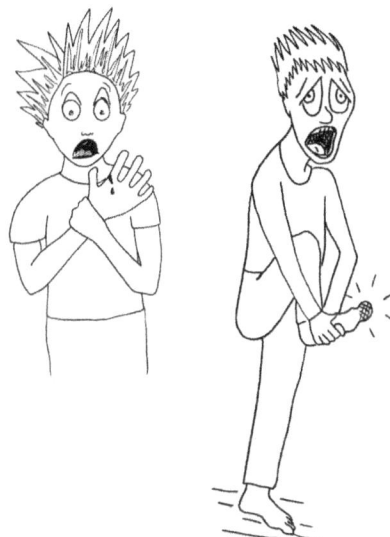

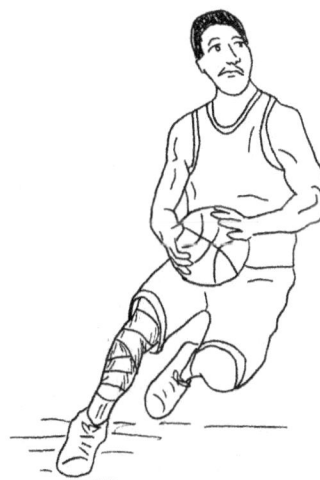

The brain works as a filter

Can you believe that the brain stores up to 500 encyclopaedias in it and filters millions of messages in a millisecond?

Imagine if you went into a supermarket and your brain had to see and know all the information that was in there – and all you wanted was milk!

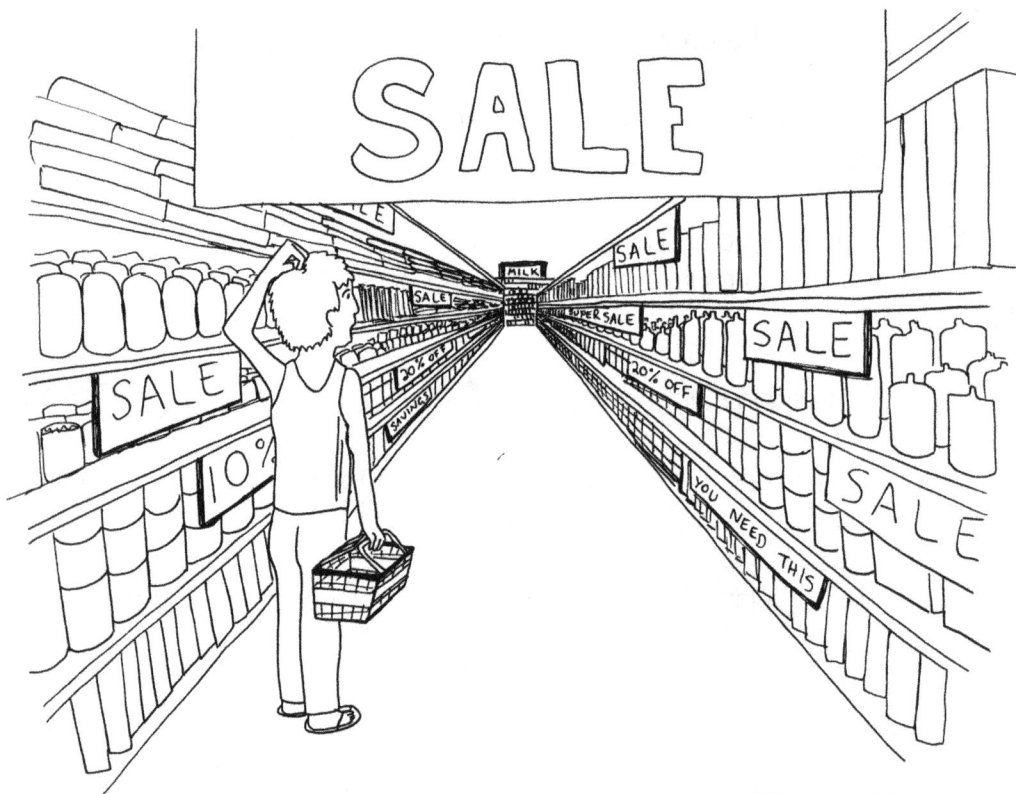

The brain is continually responding to the neurones or nerve sensors that are all throughout the body. The activation of these sensors is called nociception.

The sensors trigger messages to be sent to your brain about temperature, pressure, acidity (due to inflammation, excessive exercise or poor diet) and many other factors. Many messages are filtered at the spinal cord level. Most are being acted on automatically all the time to protect you from injuring yourself.

For instance, your neck muscles cannot stretch beyond a certain point when you unintentionally fall asleep, no matter where this might be. Stretch receptors in the neck muscles are activated because the muscles would be damaged if you stayed in such a position. The brain reacts; you wake up, and the risk of injuring your neck muscles is removed.

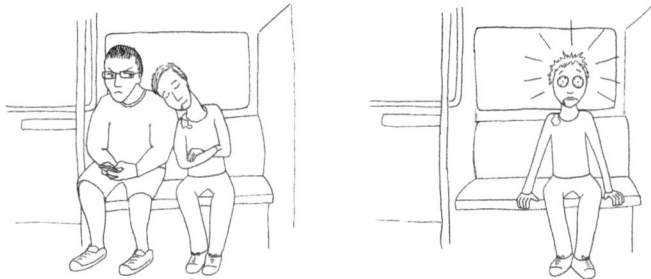

Warning system

Our sensory system is always helping us make decisions.

What is too hot or too cold? Is it safe to cross the road or not? Is this food too old to be eaten?

Lactic acid in our muscles tells us, after an intensive bout of exercise, that our muscles simply cannot contract anymore.

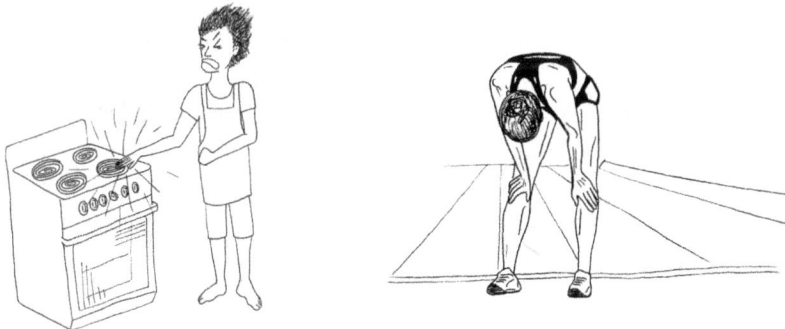

Pain sensors have a short life

The fantastic news is that the life of a nerve or pain sensor is short, only a few days. As a result, your emotional and physical reaction to pain is probably one of the most important indicators of whether an episode of pain will become a longstanding condition.

Pain is in your brain. However, provided you have been cleared by a medical practitioner, you can use exercise and positive thinking to influence how quickly your pain resolves.

💡 Points to remember

▸ Anatomical findings on radiological scans might not reveal the cause of your back pain. Many changes seen on a scan are normal age-related effects.

▸ Your health professional will be able to assess you, correlate your clinical symptoms with the scans and recommend the best solution.

▸ You are in charge of the messages that you send to your brain when you have back pain. The more positive these are, the better chance you will have of recovering from an episode and averting longstanding pain.

✓ Actions to take

▸ Do not base all decisions about how to move only on the findings of scans.

▸ You need to work with your health practitioner and possibly modify some of your daily exercises.

▸ The goal is to maintain basic fitness and keep moving as freely and confidently as you can.

Notes

11 Fitness, advanced stability and strengthening

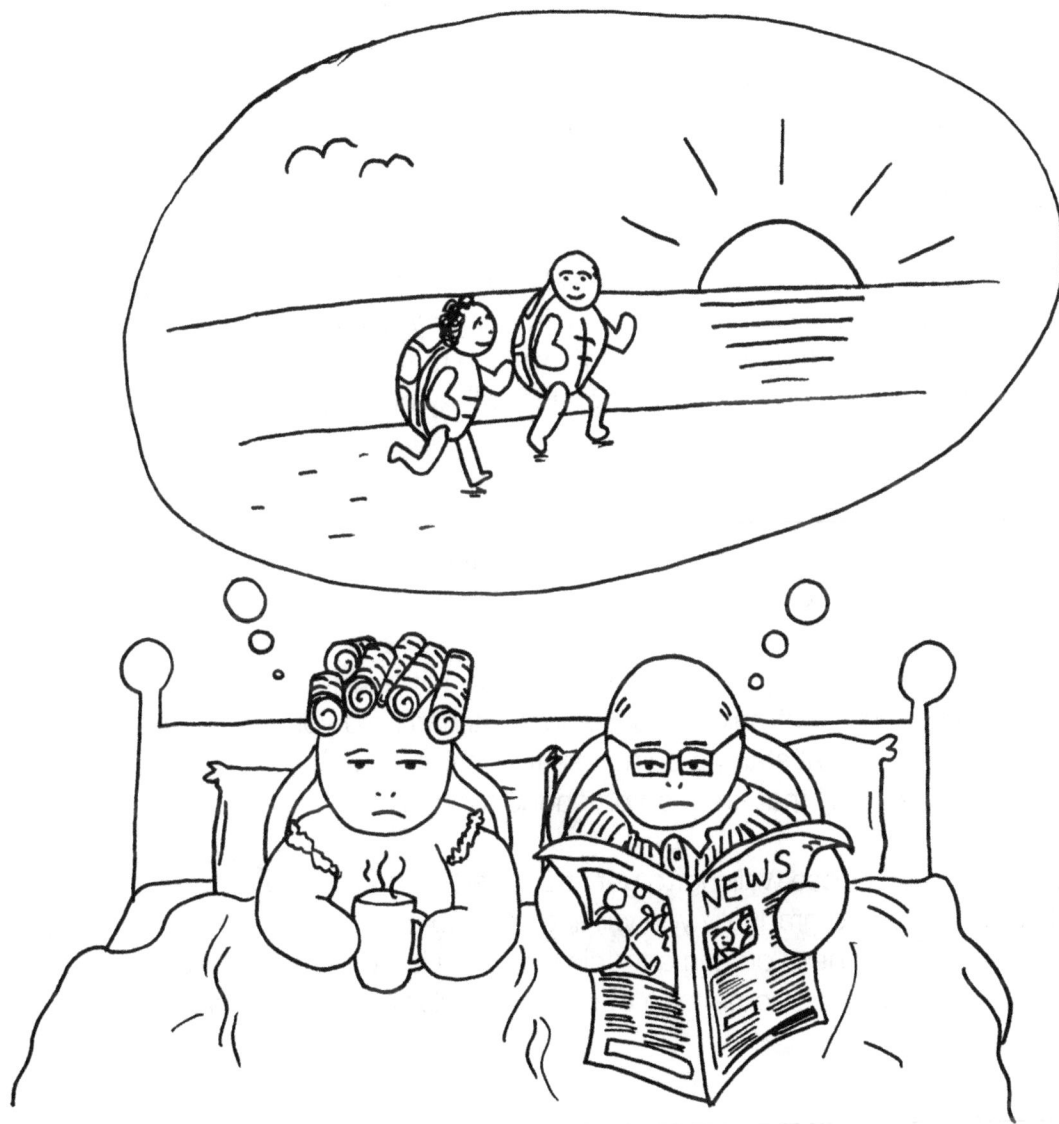

Keeping fit will help you to recover

You now understand some of the common back pain terms that you might hear. You know the stretches and stability exercises that you should be doing. The next step is to learn how to improve your overall fitness and undertake more challenging exercises using equipment.

General fitness

Your general cardiovascular fitness level greatly influences how quickly you recover from an acute episode of pain. The fitter you are, the quicker your body recovers. It is vital to choose forms of exercise that you enjoy. Many people set unrealistic expectations and then regret that they did not fulfil them.

The perfect exercise is the one that you will do.

Set realistic goals and record your progress; this will motivate you and help monitor your progress.

Return to the basics if you are recommencing a fitness program, and build up from there. Many electronic devices and apps can help you do this. A basic pedometer is a great starting point; use it to check whether you have taken the 10,000 steps a day that are recommended for basic fitness.

Suppose you choose walking to get fitter. Start with 20 to 30 minutes on alternate days and gradually you will find this too easy. Introduce hills or running up some steps when you can and this will make it more challenging and more fun. The goal is to do some form of cardiovascular fitness daily, with one day of rest per week.

Tips for improving general fitness

Here are some practical ways to increase your fitness:

▸ Do 30 minutes of aerobic exercise at least three times a week; increase this over time to five or six days.

▶ As you walk more regularly, incorporate stairs and hills to challenge yourself a little more.

▶ Run up stairs when possible. This is a great way to strengthen quads and gluteals.

▶ Do as much incidental exercise as you can. Can you get off the bus a stop earlier and walk the rest of the way to work? How often can you use the stairs instead of the lift?

Gym exercises

Try these exercises at a gym to advance your fitness further.

▶ Using a cross trainer or elliptical machine is a safe way to improve general fitness. Be aware of your core muscles; use your hands on the bar in front initially but as you get more confident, place only your fingers on the bar and this will challenge your core muscles a little more.

▶ A stationary bike can also be a good place to start.

▶ Doing a spin class would be the next progression, once you know that your back is fine after using the bike for a few weeks.

▶ Do not use a rowing machine until you have exercised for at least a few weeks with no back pain.

▶ Delay using the stepper machine until your health professional approves your doing this exercise.

Work with a health professional or personal trainer who can teach you how to use other equipment. This will also enable you to safely do more challenging resistance training.

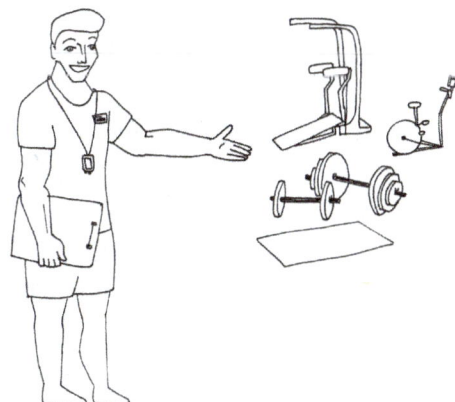

Staying motivated

Use these tips to stay motivated and to keep exercising.

▸ You could explore a new activity that is fun as well as providing you with a cardiovascular workout. Dancing would be one way.

▸ You could take a gentle yoga or tai chi class.

▸ Stay motivated by training with a friend.

▸ Use an app that records weekly exercise and shows you how much you are improving.

▸ Research shows that over-60s should exercise with a friend. If you are overweight, it is best to be supervised by a trainer. Working with others in this way improves commitment to your exercise program.

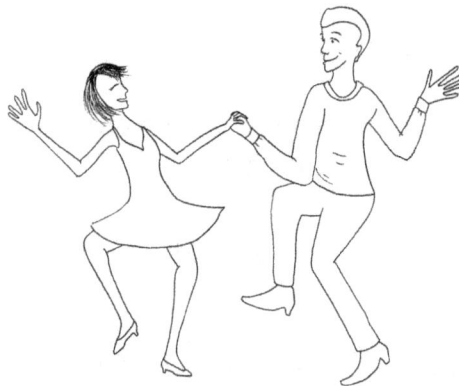

Exercise produces natural medicine

When you exercise your brain releases endorphins, opiates and other neurotransmitters. These help reduce pain and improve your overall mood and sense of well-being.

Below are three stages that you will go through until exercise becomes a routine part of your life.

Stage 1. The tough challenge

Exercising daily for the first 10 days will call for a huge physical and mental effort. Do not give up at this stage.

Stage 2. The physical phase

From 10 days to three weeks, exercising will be a little easier on the mind and body. You will go further more easily and not exert as much energy. You will be less tired on the days following exercise. But after about three weeks, the risk is that you could become bored. It is good to do something different at the end of week three to avert boredom. For instance, if walking near your home, take a different direction and find a more scenic or interesting path.

Stage 3. Positive addiction

Through weeks four, five and six, the release of natural endorphins in the brain while exercising helps us to feel healthier and happier. However, the risk at this stage is that many people start to get bored and do not persevere beyond four weeks. The goal is to take the challenge and persist.
Once you get to six weeks, you will miss exercising when you do not do it for a few days. This is a good sign that you are achieving a much better and improved level of fitness.

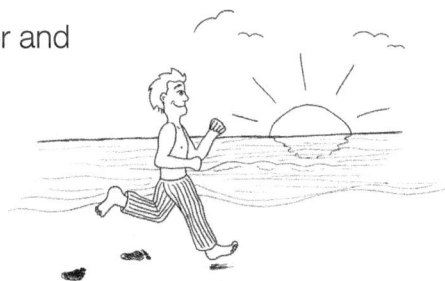

The benefits of exercising in a pool

Swimming is the fitness activity that is least stressful for the lower back. However, if you cannot or do not swim, there are many exercises that can be done in the shallow end of a pool to maintain your core strength and improve your flexibility. I have outlined some of these so that you can have fun exercising in the water. Alternatively, if you prefer to exercise in a group, doing an aquarobics class is a great place to start.

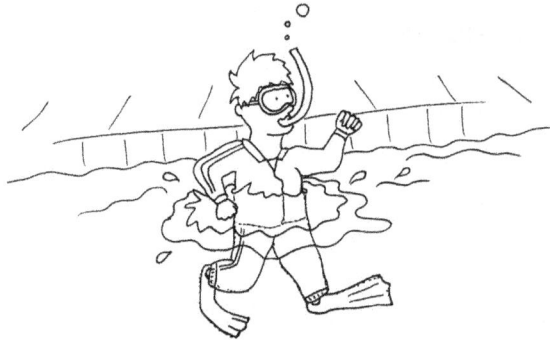

"I do feel a bit silly using these flippers and training snorkel – maybe I am doing something wrong – everybody seems to be looking"

Pool workout tips

If you can swim, try these methods of keeping fit.

▸ Invest in flippers and a kickboard. Add a training snorkel, which reduces the rotation of the lower back. With the snorkel and the flippers you can focus on breathing and on engaging core muscles as you swim. Try having the kickboard out the front, but keep it close to the top of your head, using a freestyle stroke at half-pace. This is a highly beneficial abdominal, back and

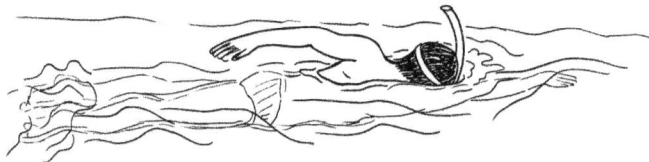

gluteal strengthening exercise, although your appearance might intrigue onlookers.

▸ If your back aches after swimming, have a coach assess the problem and teach you correct technique.

- If you do not have access to a coach, take a video film of your swimming technique and show it to your health professional. There are many apps that make this easy to do. It is usually better to let someone else identify what is causing your pain than to try and do this yourself.

- Pectoral stretches, thoracic spine extensions and better core stability will all assist if you get back pain after swimming.

Other pool exercises

If you do not swim, here are some other beneficial pool activities.

- Walk forwards and backwards in the pool with your hands by your side, palms facing the front. The water resistance will engage your core muscles.

- While walking in the water, place a kickboard under your fingertips and push it down into the water. Keep it under the water as you walk forwards and backwards; it is surprisingly hard to do. You may need to use your entire palm at first, to push the board under. Be careful that the board does not pop up out of the water.

- Hold the kickboard clear of the water with your fingertips (palm up). Be aware of your posture as you do this.

- In the deep end of the pool, even if you have not learned to swim, you could try dog-paddling, which is surprisingly challenging, or treading water on the spot.

- Use a foam belt or noodle, and tread water. This will work a lot of muscles that you might not have felt for a while.

- Try an aquarobics class. This can be challenging, but the exercises are fun and the risk to your back is usually negligible.

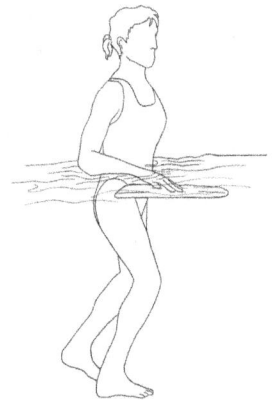

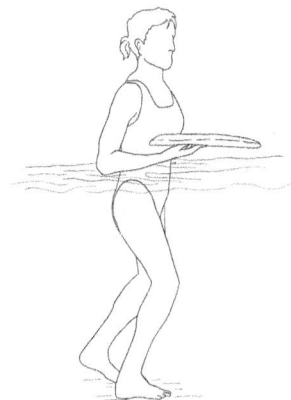

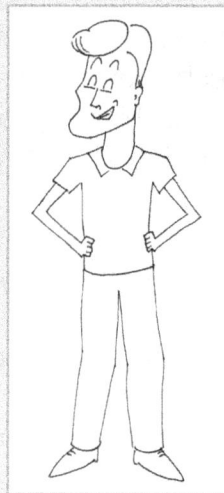

Notes from the clinic

It is vital to be motivated to keep fit.

When you are free from back pain, you can readily forget to do daily exercises.

The most important factor in overcoming your back pain in the long term is to maintain basic fitness and to do stretches and stability exercises at least three times a week.

Tips on general fitness

- *Use a pedometer to check that you take at least 10,000 steps a day.*

- *Use an app or diary in which you record weekly exercise. Get a friend involved so that you can check on each other's progress.*

- *Place your gym or exercise clothes out ready the night before. Make them visible so that it is easier to put them on, particularly if it is a cold morning.*

- *Find some friends who are also trying to maintain a regular fitness schedule.*

- *Do not think of fitness as a chore. Perhaps it is time that you tried a new activity such as dancing. You could take lessons with friends.*

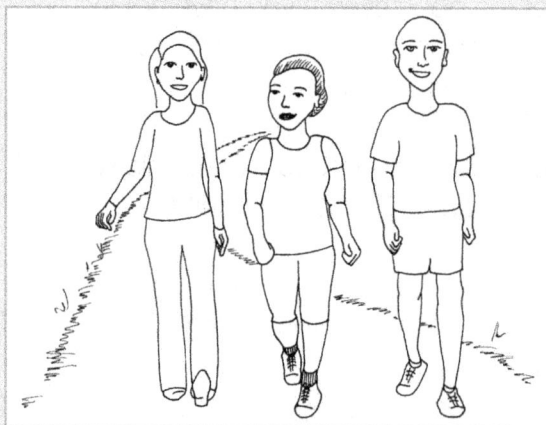

Advanced stability and strengthening with equipment

Once you have learned the basic exercises, many of which you do while lying down, you should progress to standing as soon as you can; this enables you to add resistance or weight. All day you are bending, stretching and lifting, so the goal is to be able to do this with all the correct muscles engaging automatically to support and protect your back. The following exercises are often called functional, because they replicate the movements we do in daily life.

Using exercise equipment, such as a foam beam, fitball, elasticised band or light weights, provides an extra challenge at this stage of your back pain recovery. You will have fun with some of these exercises and you will notice that your core stability, balance and overall strength are improving.

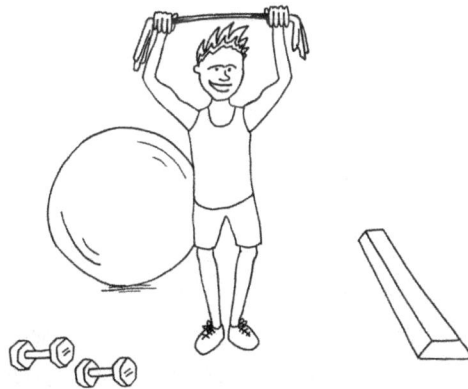

If you are not familiar with using such exercise equipment, have a physiotherapist or qualified personal trainer show you how to use them safely.

Exercise 73. The foam beam

Try standing on a foam beam or a long plank of wood and maintain your balance. Just stand in one position at first, breathe and be aware of all your core muscles without bracing. Ideally, place the beam next to a wall so that you can put your fingers on the wall until you feel more confident. Progress to transferring your weight from one foot to the other, and then walk forwards and backwards, slowly and carefully. The goal is to stand balanced on the beam, close your eyes for about five seconds, then open them. Alternate each foot in front; you will quickly note any discrepancy in the stability muscles on either side of your body.

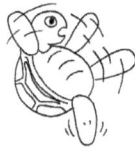

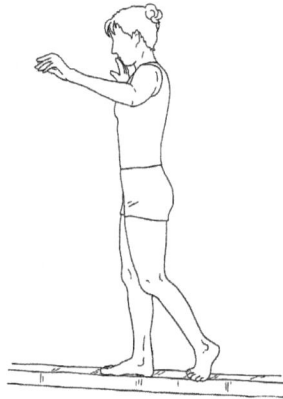

"Seriously, what will they think of next?"

If you want to have more fun with stability exercises, try walking on a beam while you are tossing a small ball. You may need to start with simply walking on the beam and doing flutter of the hand before you can handle throwing the ball. This is a great exercise if your sport calls for eye–hand co-ordination.

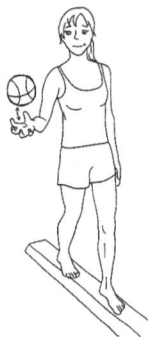

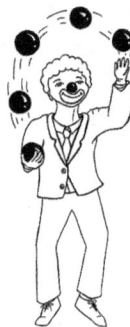

Exercise 74. Abdominal exercises using a beam

All your core stability exercises can be made more challenging by doing them on the beam.

Lie face-up along the beam. Breathe and relax your lower back. Progress to leg slides, leg drop-outs and leg floats. Take care not to overarch your back; maintain contact with

the beam. To make this exercise even more challenging, raise your arms in the air at a right-angle to the ground and repeat all of your leg exercises (see Chapter 6 for detailed descriptions of these exercises).

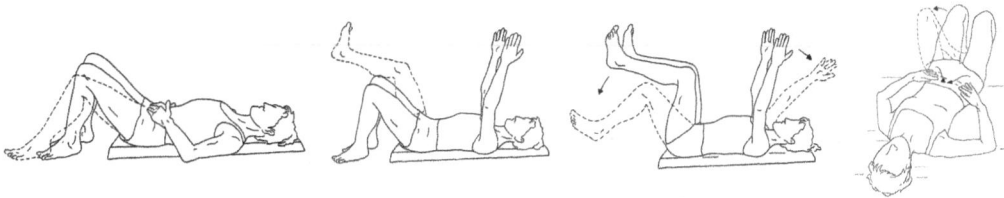

Exercise 75. Flutter while sitting on an exercise ball

Place your hands behind you on an exercise ball as you sit on the ball. Once you feel balanced, take your hands off the ball and maintain your posture. Try to flutter one hand while you gently do a pelvic tilt forwards and backwards a few times.

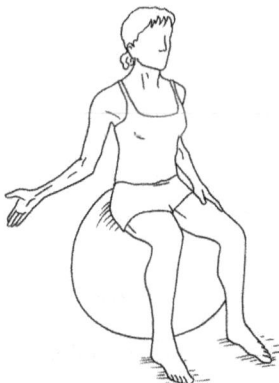

Exercise 76. Lower abdominals

On all fours, rest your head and shoulders on an exercise ball. Touch your fingers onto the ground on either side, for stability. Let your abdomen relax completely. Engage your pelvic floor and lower abdominals. Think of lifting one knee and only slightly initiate this movement. You will feel your core muscles engage. Repeat this on the other leg. Place your hands on the ball and try to achieve the same movement of lifting each knee just slightly. Repeat four or five times on each leg.

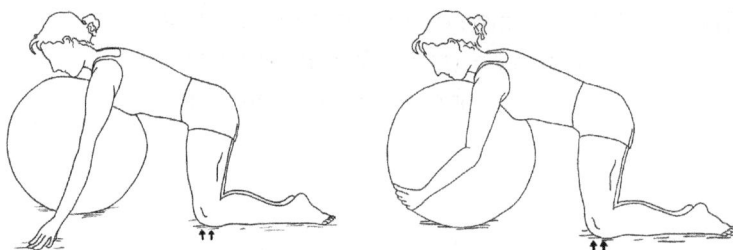

Exercise 77. Lower abdominals with hip extension

Start this exercise with your fingers touching the ground while resting head and shoulders on the exercise ball. Engage your lower abdominals and then slide one leg out behind. Repeat on each leg and try not to drop too far laterally into the hip. Once you feel confident that you can do this easily, progress to holding the ball as you extend the leg. The advanced progression is to keep your hands on the ball and lift the leg off the ground while it is extended. Repeat four or five times for each leg.

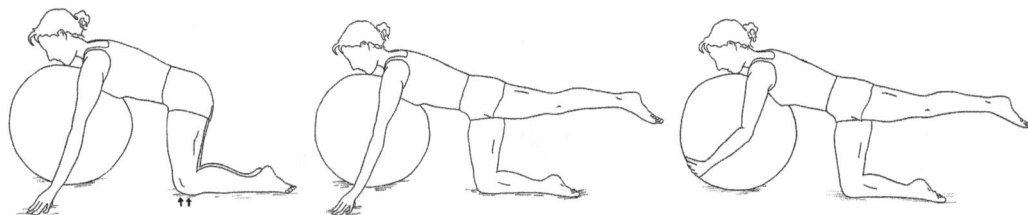

Exercise 78. Lying on your back, ball above the head

While lying on your back, take the exercise ball in your finger-tips and hold it above you at chest level. Breathe in, and as you exhale, take the ball 20–30 degrees above your head. This is an excellent exercise for engaging your core muscles. Be sure to not let your back overarch, and do not brace your abdominals. Once you can repeat this 10 times and you know it is not causing pain in your lower back, try taking the ball 4 or 5 times approximately 20–30 degrees to each side. This will start to engage your oblique abdominal muscles.

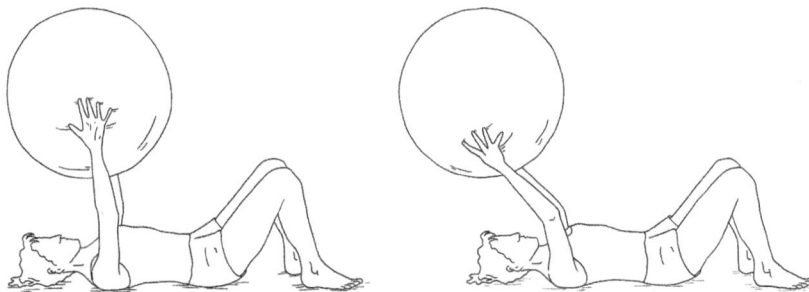

Exercise 79. Strengthening gluteals

Sit on the exercise ball. Keep your hands on the ball as you roll down until the ball is supporting the back of your shoulder-blades, head and neck. Slightly tuck your chin in. Cross your arms so that your hands are on opposite shoulders, and use your gluteal muscles to lift your pelvis. You can stay close to the ground at first, but if your back feels fine, lift the pelvis higher. Take care not to hyperextend; that is, do not overarch your back.

To progress this exercise, straighten your arms out to the side, maintaining your balance. Drop the pelvis lower as you place your arms on opposite shoulders. Now lift the pelvis again and outstretch the arms. Repeat 10 times if you can.

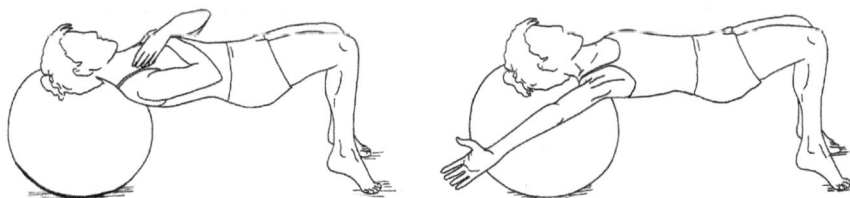

Exercise 80. Strengthening abdominals without the sit-up

Lie on your back and rest your feet over the exercise ball. Imagine that there is a feather under your calf muscle. Breathe in; as you exhale, lift your shin bone just a little, as if lessening the weight on the feather. This is an excellent alternative for toning all of your abdominals if sit-ups hurt your neck or back.

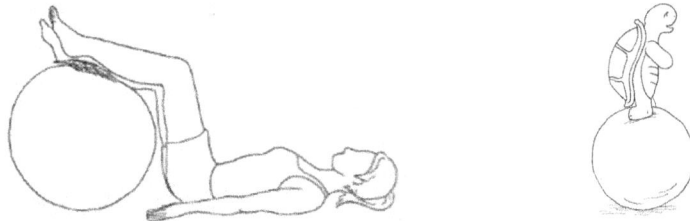

Exercise 81. Lower back release

Lie on your back with legs resting over the exercise ball. Keep your arms outstretched to the sides. Let the ball roll to one direction approximately 30 degrees; return to the midline and repeat to the other side. This should feel relaxing on your lower back, with no pain. This exercise helps you become more confident about rotating the lower back again, if you have been avoiding that movement.

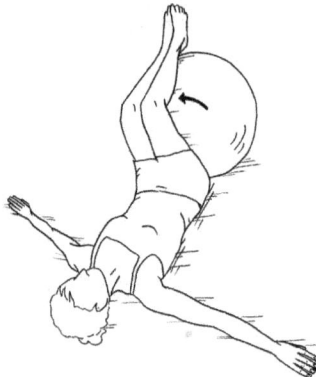

Exercises using an elastic band

You can buy elastic bands from your health professional or from an exercise equipment shop.

Start with the easiest band; progress to the next level (a band with more tension) only when you can do two sets of eight repetitions with the easier band.

Exercise 82. Triceps and mid back

Tie a band around a door handle. Hold the ends of the band in each hand and start with the elbows bent. Breathe in; as you exhale, straighten your arms down by each side. Control the tension in the band as you return to the start position. Repeat six to eight times. Slightly flex your knees so as to not overextend your lower back.

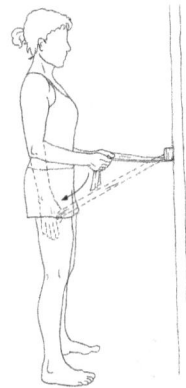

Exercise 83. Lateral hip stability

Place a band under your feet. Cross the band and hold the ends in each hand. Breathe in; as you step in one direction, maintain stability in your pelvis and hips. As you exhale, return to the midline. Do eight steps, alternating between sides on each step. Keep knees slightly flexed. You might need to start with one or two repetitions only, and build up to eight.

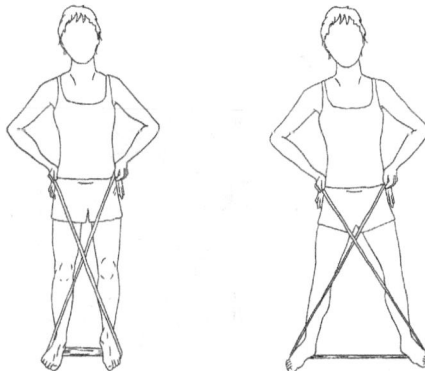

Exercise 84. Biceps curl with sideways squats

Place the band under each foot. Step to the side; adopt a partial squat position at the same time as curling the biceps. Stand tall when you return to the midline. Then squat in the same way as you move to the opposite side, and do a biceps curl again.

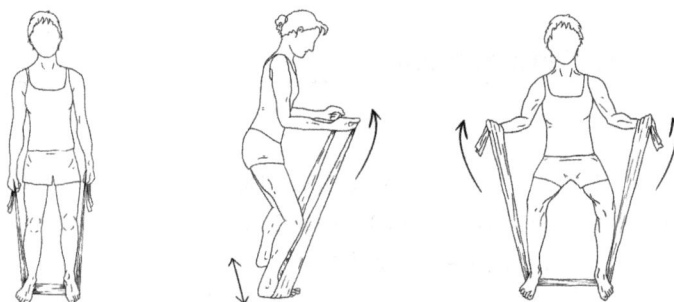

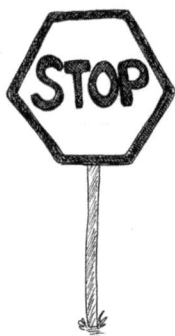

The goal is to regain normal movement

Do not progress to any of the following exercises until you are confident you can flex easily again.

You might be overprotecting your back before you lift anything, in case your back locks. If so, this will increase stiffness throughout your body. Your goal is to move as normally as possible to return your back muscles to engaging automatically.

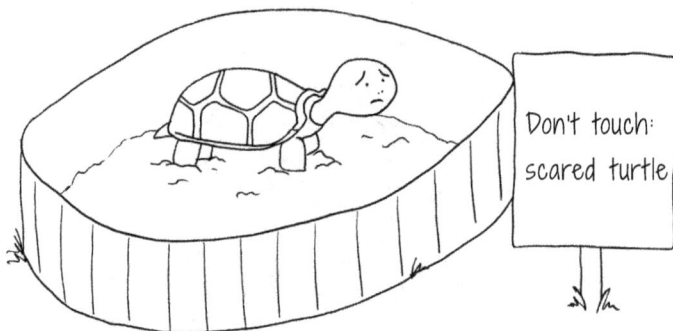

Don't touch: scared turtle

When your job requires lifting

After you have experienced an acute episode of back pain, your goal is to return to work and normal everyday activities as soon as your pain is manageable and you are moving more freely. However, it is important not to be stoic and not to return too soon, while you still have pain, as this will delay your recovery. The goal is to find out why you hurt yourself and avert a recurrence.

These are some of the manoevres that incur the highest risk of back injury:

▶ lifting with straight knees

▶ lifting and carrying an object close to the ground and placing it down again, particuarly if you need to stretch well forward in the process, and

▶ carrying a heavy weight on one shoulder and putting it down; particularly if you need to do this repetitively.

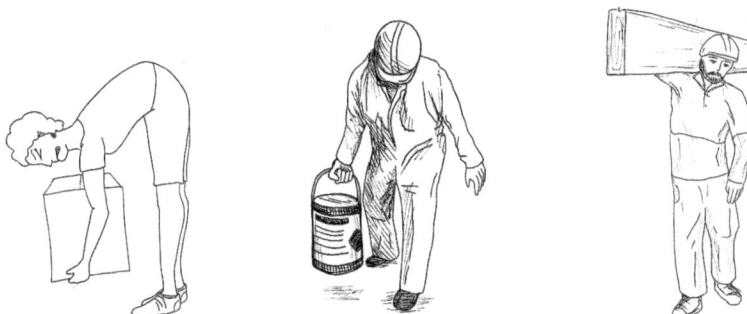

Helpful lifting tips

Before lifting, consider what you are about to lift. This is not always possible, particularly if you need to lift quickly and repetitively at work, but this is the ideal. The technique you use will depend on the weight you are lifting and the type of lift required. Assess the object you plan to lift and decide whether you need to keep it close to the ground or take it above your head.

All lifting involves varying flexibility of your hips, knees, back and shoulders. But for all lifting, excellent core awareness and strength will reduce your risk of injury.

If you have injured your back by lifting, take a photo of your workplace so that your health professional can advise you and design an exercise program to reduce your risk of injury at work.

Basic guidelines for lifting correctly

Keep these points in mind before you lift any heavy weight:

▶ Have the object to be lifted in front of you, as close to your body as possible.

▶ Breathe in; as you breathe out, engage your pelvic floor and core muscles before you lift. The heavier the object, the more you will need to engage these muscles in advance.

▶ Use your leg muscles, gluteal muscles and arm muscles to do most of the work of lifting.

▶ If you need to put the object down to either side or behind you, do not twist your body but turn to face where you want to place the object before you start to put it down.

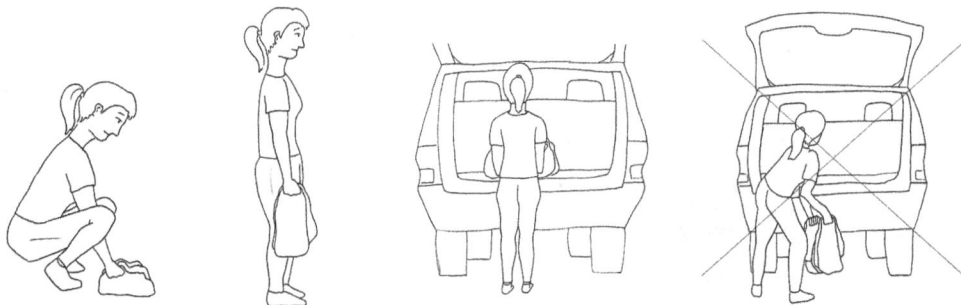

📖 *Notes from the clinic*

Do not do a full squat every time you lift anything or you might strain your knees.

A patient with a lower back injury was doing her exercises at home and reviewing progress with me regularly. One knee had swollen but she did not know why. I discovered that her knee pain was caused by her adopting an extreme deep squat position not only for lifting but every time she bent forward: putting on shoes, going to low drawers, opening the oven door, picking up a child. She had taken too literally my advice to keep her back straight and bend the knees when she lifted.

This client was also hypermobile, which meant that she could fully squat easily. She needed to stop going into a deep squat every time she lifted something. The swelling of her knee resolved quite quickly once she stopped overthinking about the way to lift and started bending and moving more normally. I designed some new exercises to give her the confidence to bend again. Her knee pain did not return and her back pain continued to resolve.

Regain the confidence to bend again

⚠️ **CAUTION:** If you have lost the confidence to bend, try this gentle movement, but do not do this when you have back pain. The time to do it is when you are free from pain.

Roll down the wall: Stand with your back resting against a wall. Keep your heels away from the wall, with your knees slightly bent. Gently start to let your head curl forward and release and bend your spine slowly downwards until you are flexed as far as you can go. Let your hands relax on the floor and then start at the base of your spine and slowly curl up and return to a standing position. If you can do this without pain, reverse the movement. Start with your hands on the floor and then gradually curl back up into a standing position again.

Once you can roll down the wall without pain, you can progress to the following exercises, which require bending and flexing more freely and confidently.

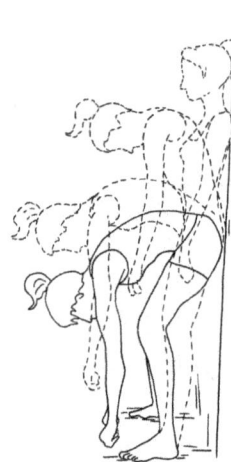

Exercise 85. Pick up paper

Take two pieces of A4 paper, one in each hand and follow this sequence:

▸ With your right hand, place one sheet just in front of your right foot.

▸ With your left hand, place the sheet of paper in front of your left foot with the top of the paper about 10 centimetres further forward than where the top of the paper was on the right side.

▸ Place your left foot forward onto the paper.

▸ With your right hand, pick up the piece of paper on the right and move it forward about 20 centimetres. (The challenge is to take this step with the right leg off the ground.)

▸ Repeat this sequence, moving a little further forward each time; the goal is to do this at least three to five times with each leg.

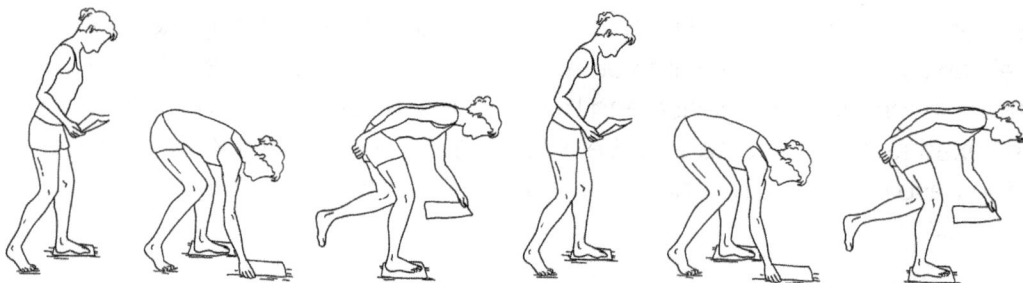

The goal of this fun exercise is to get you to stop overthinking when you go to bend, even when lifting a light object.

⚠ **CAUTION:** If you feel the slightest twinge in your back, you are not ready to do this sequence. Try it again in a few weeks.

Exercise 86. Roll-downs

⚠ **CAUTION:** You must be able to do a wall roll-down with no pain before you try this exercise.

Sit-ups can aggravate pain in the neck or back. Supported roll-downs are a safe alternative way to maintain strength through the full range of the spine.

Tie an elasticised band onto a door handle. Sit on the floor with the end of the band in each hand. Try not to use your arms; tuck in your chin as you curl and roll backwards to the ground. Use the band to help lift your body up again.

Start with only three or four repetitions. When you know this exercise is not aggravating your back pain, you can easily increase this to 10 repetitions.

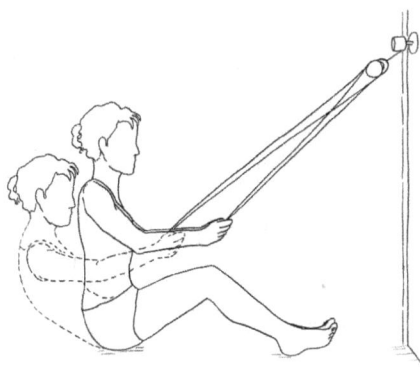

If you attend a gym, look for a strong strap secured to a bar or roof beam. Most gyms have one. It is a useful piece of equipment with which to do a controlled roll-down.

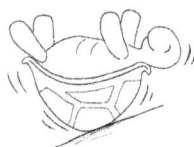

"I find this really easy"

Using light weights for strengthening

When you have had longstanding back pain, often you have lost strength in your upper body and lower body. Using weights can help you to regain the strength and confidence to move more freely and confidently again.

Begin with light weights; 1.5 kilograms is an ideal starting point. Increase this to 2.0 kilograms once you can do two sets of eight repetitions. Progress by half a kilogram at a time. Give yourself a few weeks to be sure that your back is coping with the extra weight before you add more kilograms.

Exercise 87. Arm raises plus weights

While standing in a slight squat position, with a light weight in each hand (start with 1.0 or 1.5 kilos), raise the arm above your head. Alternate arms; start with five raises on each side and progress to 10.

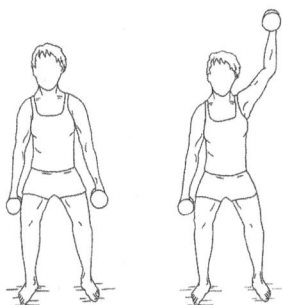

Exercise 88. Arm raises on an exercise ball, with weights

Sit on the exercise ball, with a light weight in each hand (1.0 or 1.5 kilograms). Think of standing, so that your core is engaged. Raise one weight above your head and lower it. Alternate arms; do six to eight repetitions on each side. Keep the weight close to your body. Start with palms facing your legs, then rotate the hand as you lift so that the palm is at the front when your arm is above your head.

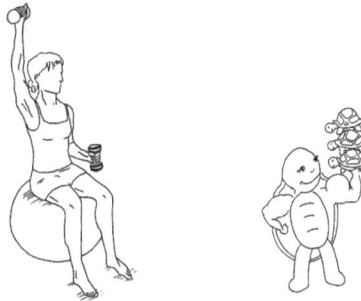

Exercise 89. Strengthening gluteals and quadriceps

Hold a cylindrical weight with fingertips; start with 2.5 kilograms. Stand as
naturally as possible and move as if to sit on a chair or stool behind you. Stop
just short of the chair, and return to standing. As you stand, be conscious
of your gluteals doing the work. You will notice that you need to use your
quadriceps, gluteals and your core muscles if you are doing the exercise
correctly. Try to keep your weight on your heels. Repeat eight to twelve times.

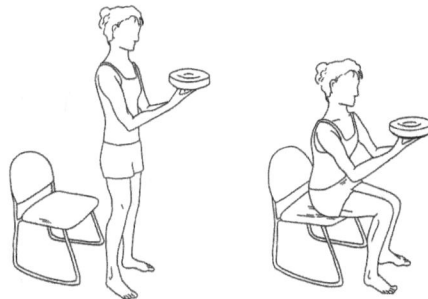

Exercise 90. Lifting a bar to raise confidence

⚠ **CAUTION:** Consult your health professional before doing this exercise. If you
do not have an expert to guide you, start the exercise with a light bar such as
a broomstick. This will get you moving and lifting in a more natural manner, and
you can work up to using a weighted bar.

Follow this sequence:

▸ Place both hands on a bar on the floor, and adopt a squatting position.

▸ Stand with your feet turned outwards, placed slightly wider than your hips.

- ▸ Keep your knees aligned with your feet and make sure that your weight is on your heels.

- ▸ Look ahead; lift the bar as you move to a standing position, keeping the bar close to the body.

- ▸ While standing, bend your elbows to rotate the bar so that it is at shoulder height.

- ▸ Still looking ahead, place the bar on the floor again.

This exercise should be done in a smooth, flowing movement. The goal is to do two sets of eight to ten repetitions.

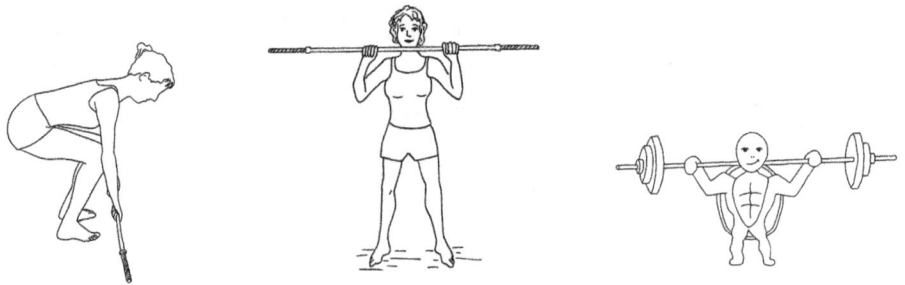

For the best long-term results, consult an expert

If you have managed all the exercises including those in this chapter, well done, but now is not the time to stop. Once you have reached a plateau with your strengthening, it is time to consult a health or exercise professional to learn more challenging exercises than those covered to this point. You are now ready to have a program designed for your way of life, your work or your sporting needs. A trainer will also provide helpful tips on how to stay motivated and keep fit each day. But remember, no exercise should cause pain in your back; pace yourself and do not be too ambitious.

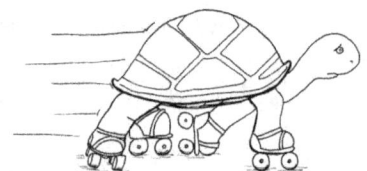

SUMMARY OF ADVANCED STABILITY EXERCISES

Using a foam beam

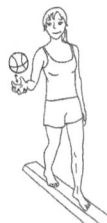

73

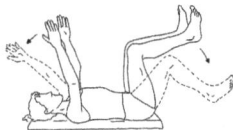

74

Using a fitball

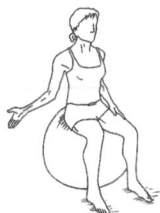

75

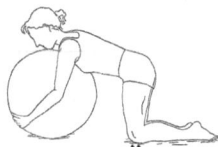

76

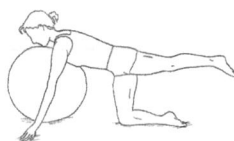

77

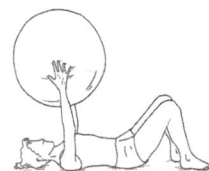

78

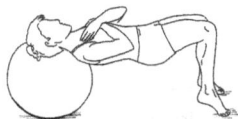

79

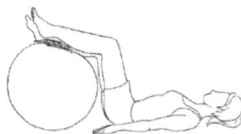

80

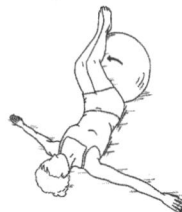

81

Using an elasticised band

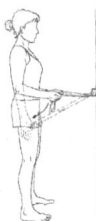

82

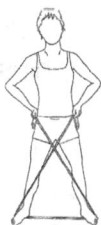

83

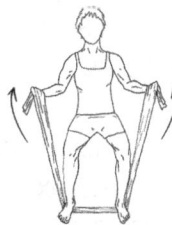

84

Exercises to regain flexing confidence

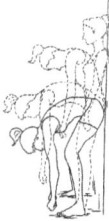 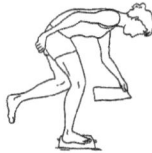 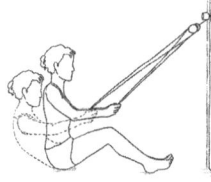

Rolling down the wall   85   86

Using weights

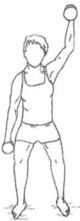 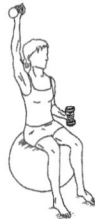 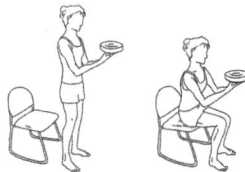 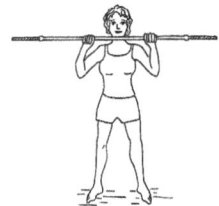

87   88   89   90

💡 Points to remember

▸ You need to improve your general fitness to overcome back pain in the long term. Some daily cardiovascular activity, for about 30 minutes, is the ideal.

▸ You need to have realistic goals. Know your starting point and build up gradually. Stay motivated by recording your goals using an app or in a diary.

▸ Understand that your challenge is to maintain your fitness program beyond four weeks until you reach six weeks. After that, exercising usually becomes automatic and enjoyable as the "happy" endorphins are released.

▸ You have learned a lot of new exercises with equipment that you can use at home. Once you can do the exercises easily, consult an exercise or health professional to progress your exercises so that they match your life, work or sporting needs.

✓≡ Actions to take

▶ Add incidental exercise when you can.

▶ Take the stairs not the lift.

▶ Park the car a little further away from your destination.

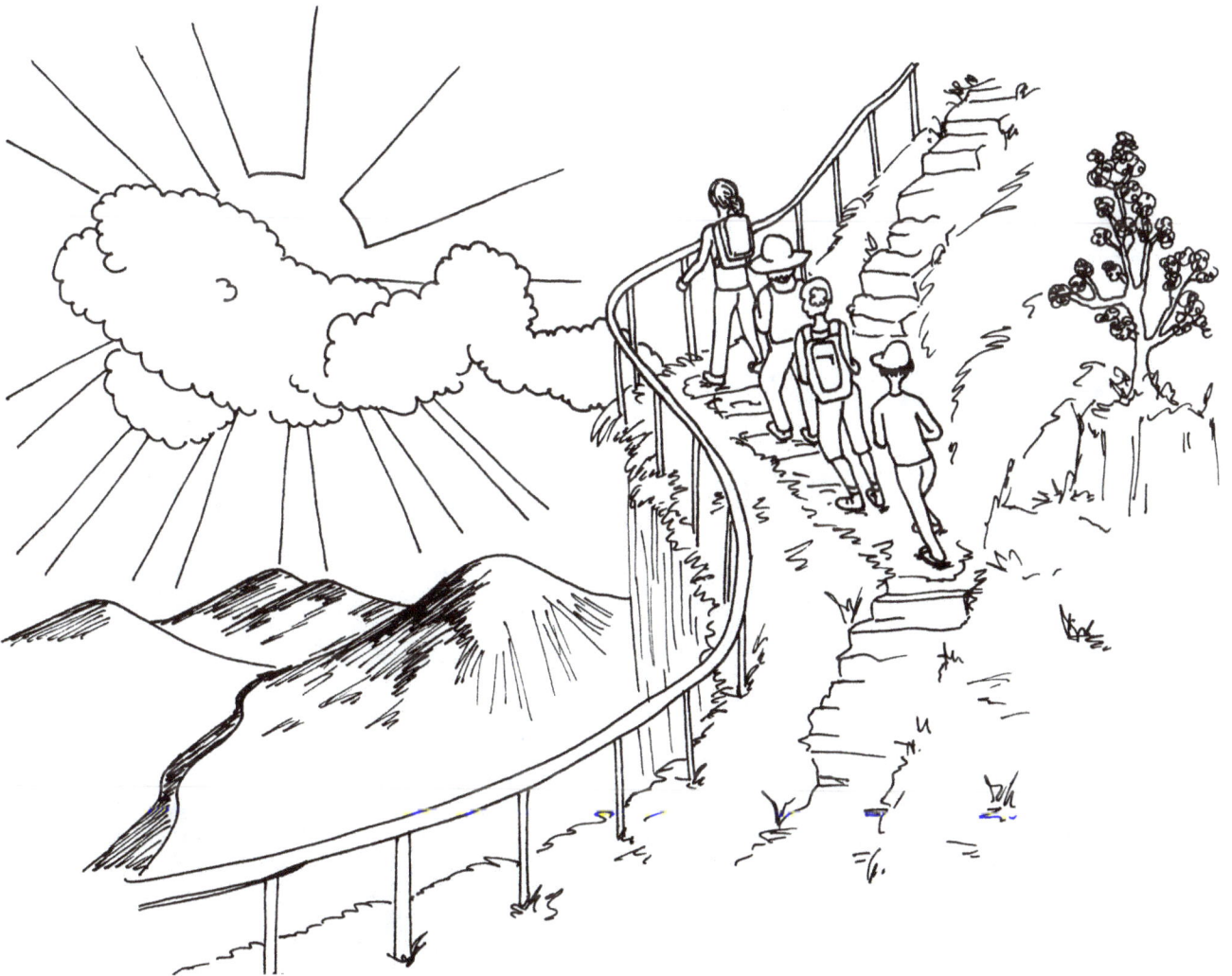

Notes

12 Reviewing the back story

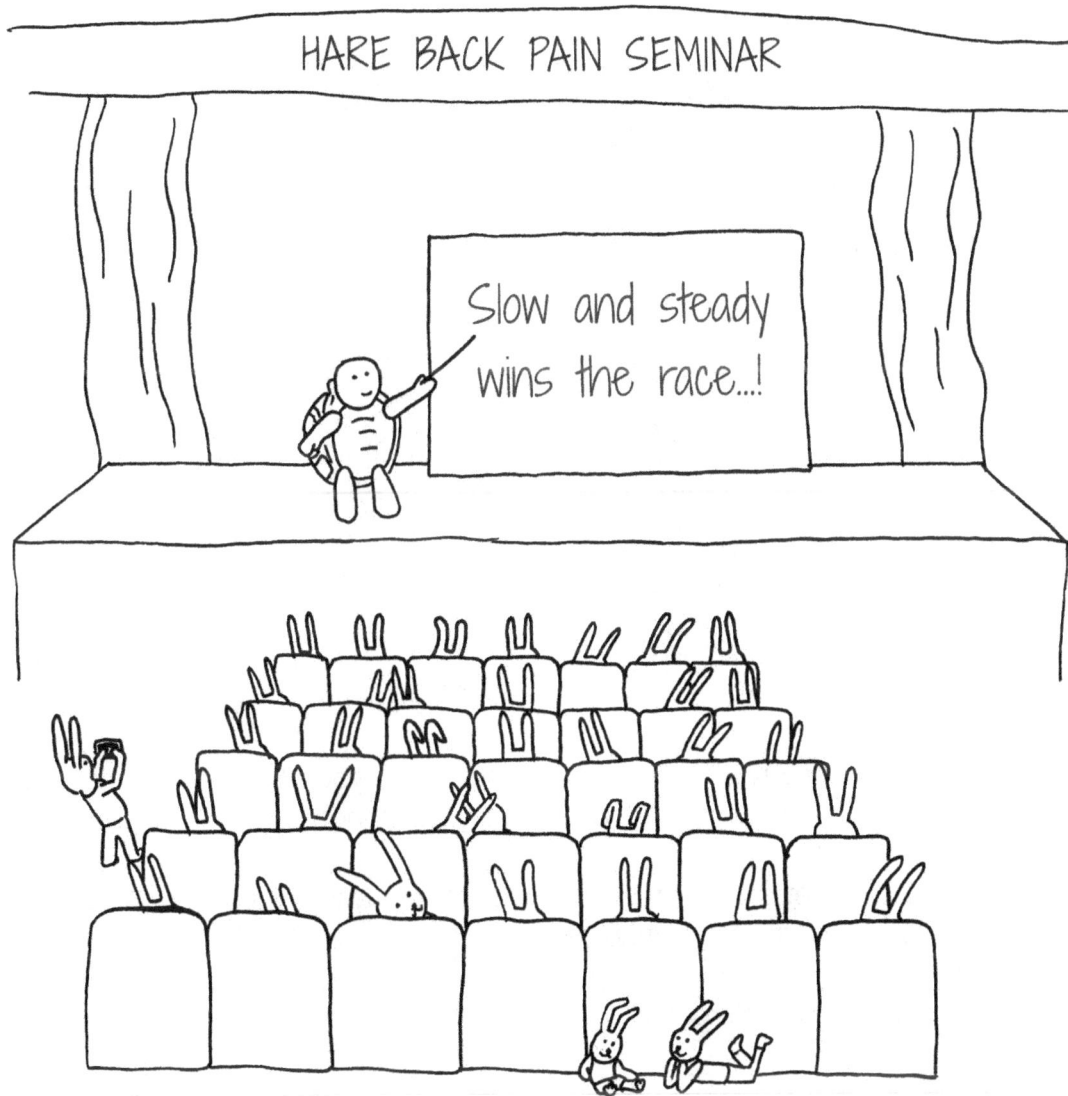

Looking after your back in the long term

You now have all the information you need on how to move, think and react a little differently when dealing with back pain.

It is possible that you will have a setback, a niggle, a feeling that your back is going to lock, or a recurrence of back pain; but you now know how to manage these.

Embrace pain as your friend

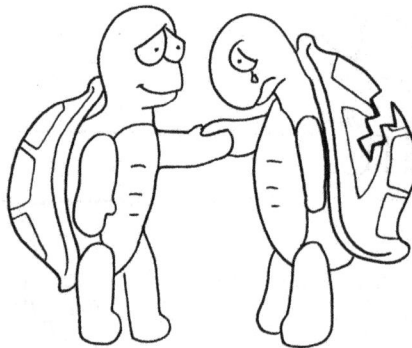

Seeing pain as a friend might seem at odds with how you feel when in pain; but this is your goal, to view pain as an opportunity to change your lifestyle.

Remember, pain is setting off your alarm system and telling you that your body is at risk. Pain prompts you to ask yourself:

▶ Have I let my fitness go recently?

▶ Have I gone back to my old postural habits?

▶ What was I doing during the past few days that might have caused this to happen?

Many patients tell me that they were no longer feeling back pain, so they stopped doing stretching and core exercises. I hear this too often from patients I have not seen for some time.

Stop acute pain from becoming chronic

Here are three steps you can take to ease pain and avert longer term problems.

Step 1. Calm your alarm system

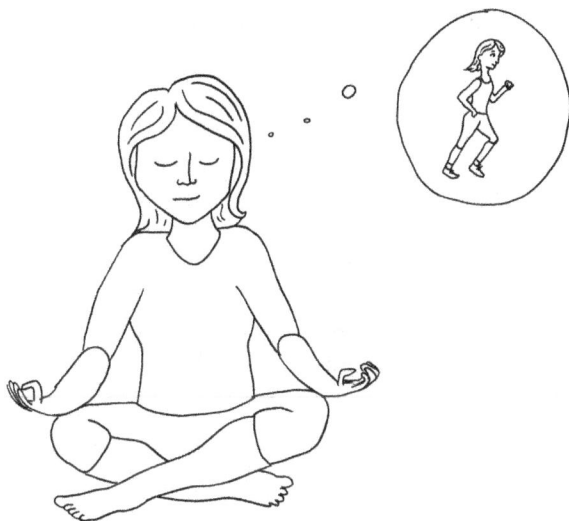

Remember not to overreact when you feel that pain or tightness in your back is returning. If possible, step away from what you are doing and spend some time, preferably alone, to focus on your breathing. As you feel your muscles starting to relax, visualise yourself moving normally again.

Step 2. Move normally as soon as you can

Use a brace for a few days if it helps you to move more confidently and freely. Take the brace off as you commence your exercises again.

Step 3. Relax and stretch the tight muscles

Do upper limb neural exercises then those for the lower limbs; add the basic core exercises. Progress to stretching your hip flexors and adductors; start these while standing, as soon as your pain level and flexibility permit.

The following exercises are particularly helpful if you are not experiencing pain but your back feels "out" or you can sense that it is starting to lock. This is usually because some muscles are in protective spasm. By relaxing these first, you will then be able to do your core exercises more easily.

Daily preventive exercise routine

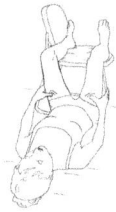

6. Relax the hip flexors

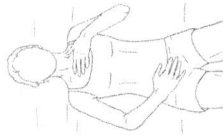

9. Relax the neck and shoulders and lower back muscles

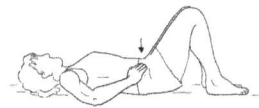

10. Engage the pelvic floor muscles

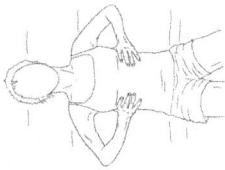

11. Diaphram breathing

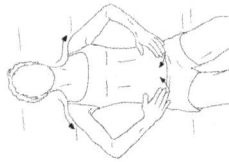

12. Engage transverse abdominus

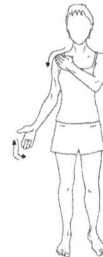

16. Flutter to automate the engaging of the core muscles

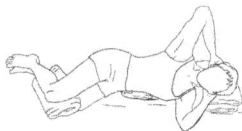

4. Start some gentle upper limb neural exercises

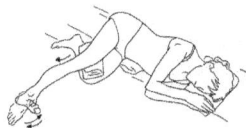

3. Providing it does not aggravate your pain commence the lower limb neural glides

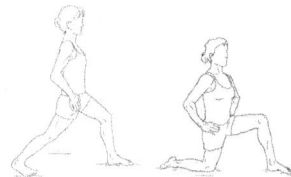

47 and 49. Try a hip flexor stretch either while standing or kneeling

For detailed descriptions of these exercises refer to Chapter 4, Chapter 6 and Chapter 7. Progress to the more challenging core stability exercises and stretches once you have recovered from the acute pain. See Appendix 2 for summaries of the exercises.

Additional tips

It is fine to take medication to ease your pain. Having a warm bath or a massage will help you to handle acute pain. Reducing pain will enable you to move more freely and normally. But always seek help from a medical professional if your pain is greater than eight out of ten, if you have severe leg pain or night pain, or if your symptoms have not settled within a few days of applying the active approach set out in this book.

Stop your pain before it starts

Prevention is crucial. Once you are moving normally again, see your health professional for a preventive check-up. Do this regularly.

No serious athlete would go longer than four to six weeks without having a coach review their exercise regime or sporting technique. Your health professional will bring you up to date with the latest research and see whether you might have strayed from good technique and form and introduced what I call "exercise innovations" into your daily regime. A review also enables a check on your current work and posture habits.

If you look after your fitness, health and daily postural habits, and keep your sense of humour, you definitely will start to move more freely and confidently again.

From professional practice and personal experience, I can assure you that overcoming back pain is indeed possible.

✏️ Notes

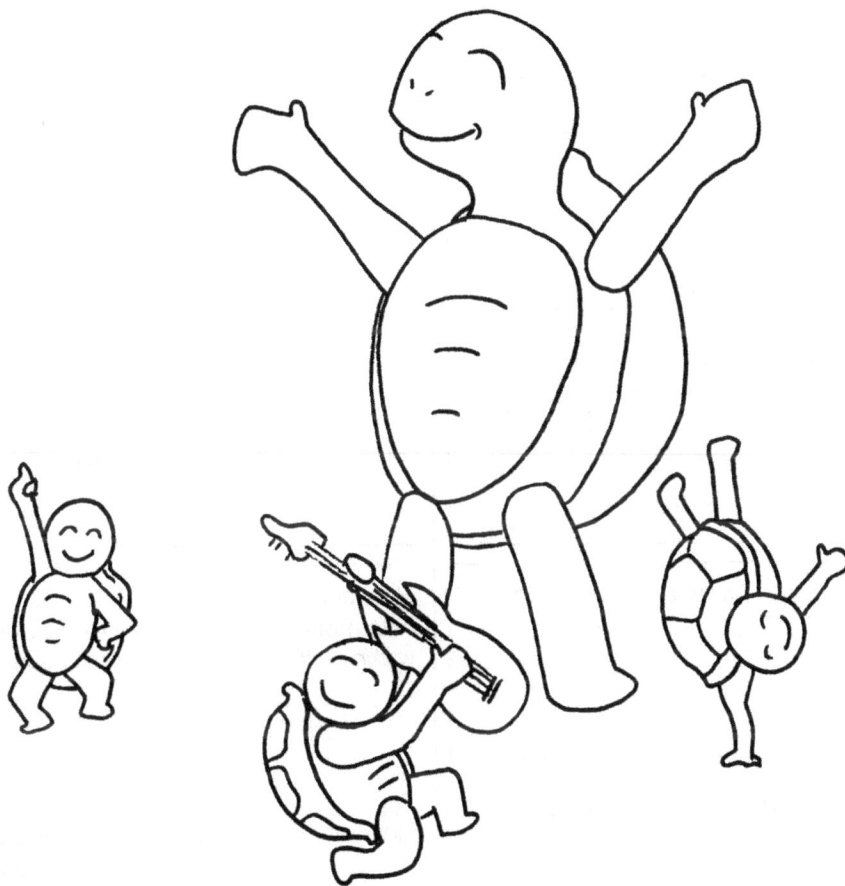

APPENDIX I

SELF ASSESSMENT 1

DATE _____

What words and phrases do I use to describe my back pain?	What more positive and active words will I now use when referring to my back?
How have I restricted my lifestyle due to pain?	What hobbies or physical activities would I like to return to?
How can I improve my general health? *(for example, diet, stress levels or work–life balance)*	What is my current fitness level? ☐ Poor ☐ Recreationally fit ☐ Excellent
If you marked poor – what exercise would you do?	How could I improve my fitness? What will help motivate me to exercise? *(for example, walking with a friend, or using an exercise app)*
I think the reason I have back pain is… My current pain score most days is: /10 On a good day: /10 On a challenging day: /10 *0 = no pain 10 = severe*	How many times per week can I realistically achieve this? *(I will record when I am achieving this at six weeks)*

My goals: Fitness (for example, walking twice a week)

Functional goal (for example, carrying the shopping)

Thoughts

Other

SELF ASSESSMENT 2: SIX WEEK PROGRESS *(Suggest that you copy a few of these pages to record your progress)*

If you get another acute episode, work your way through this and you will find you will recover much more quickly.   **DATE** _____

General fitness: Each week I am currently achieving:

Habits: I am more aware of my overall posture when I am walking, sitting and standing. The cue that is working best for me is:

My current pain score is: Good day   /10   Challenging day   /10

To decrease this score even further I need to:

-
-
-

The strategies that are helping me most when I feel a twinge of pain are: *(for example, breathing exercises, muscle meditation)*

-
-
-

The exercises I like the most that help my back are: *(for example stretches, stability)*

-
-
-

The exercises and activities that aggravate my back pain are:

-
-
-

The ways I modify this are:

APPENDIX II

SUMMARY OF ALL EXERCISES

Below is a summary of all of the exercises covered in this book, with page numbers for easy reference. I suggest that you circle the exercises that you have found to be most helpful and cross out the ones that you have found less beneficial. After a while you should be able to run through your own preferred routine with only a quick reference to your summary.

CHAPTER 4. Neural exercises and relaxing the hip flexors

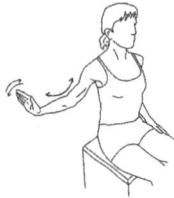

1. p48

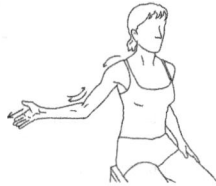

2. p49

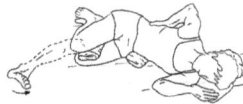

3. p51

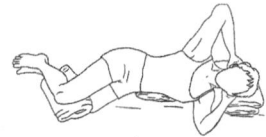

4. p51

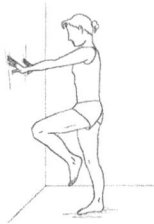

5. p52

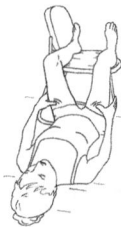

6. p56

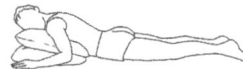

7. p57

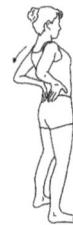

8. p58

CHAPTER 6. Core stability exercises

Level 1. Lying supine plus flutter and arm raise

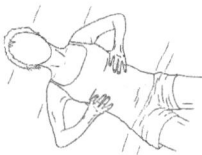

9. p94

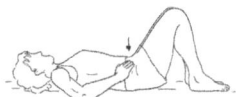

10. p95

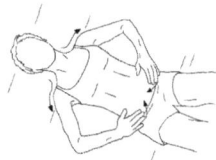

11. p95

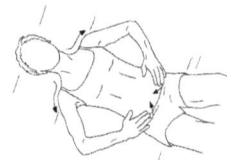

12. p96

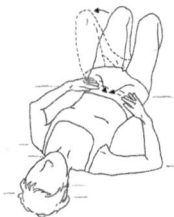

13. p96

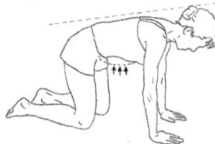

14. p97

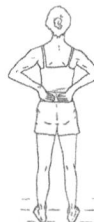

15. p98

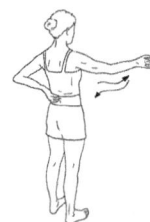

16. p99

Stability progressions
Level 2. Supine stability using the arms and legs

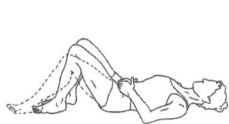

17. p99

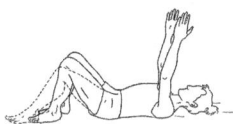

18. p100

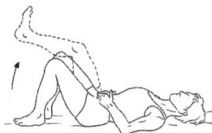

19. p100

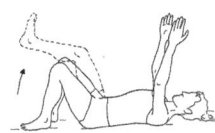

20. p101

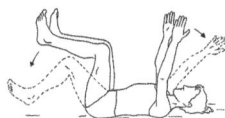

21. p101

Prone stability

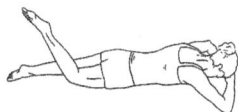

22. p102

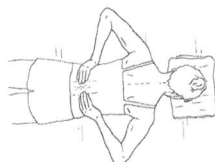

23. p102

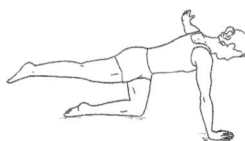

24. p103

Hip stability

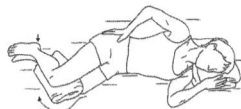

25. p106

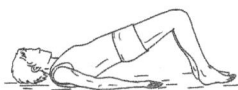

26. p107

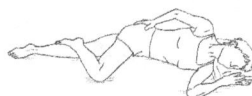

27. p108

Intermediate stability and strengthening

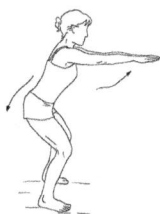

28. p108

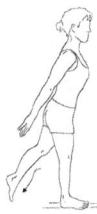

29. p109

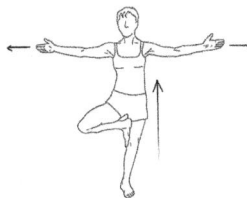

30. p109

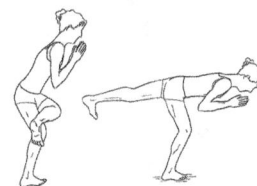

31. p110

CHAPTER 7. Stretches for the back, hips and legs

Easy

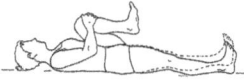

32. p117

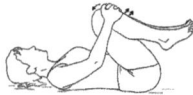

33. p117

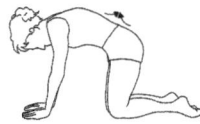

34. p118

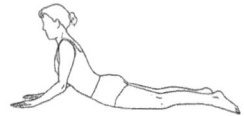

35. p118

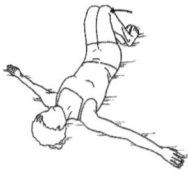

36. p119

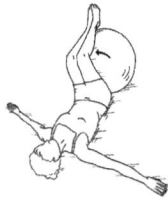

37. p120

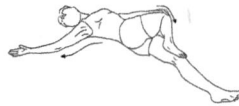

38. p120

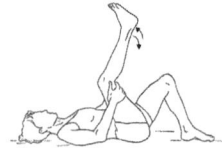

39. p125

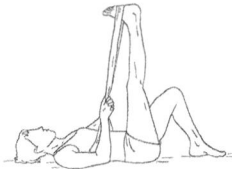

40. p126

Intermediate and advanced

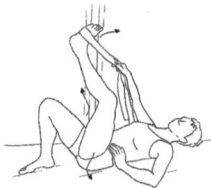

41. p127

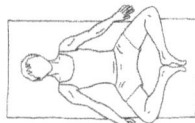

42. p129

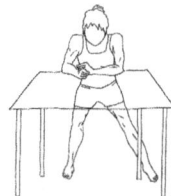

43. p129

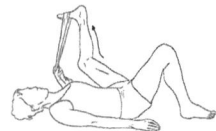

44. p130

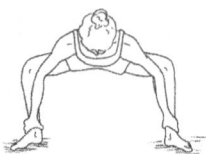

45. p130

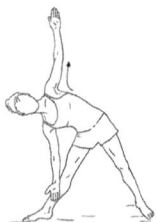

46. p131

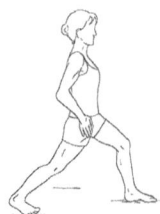

47. p132

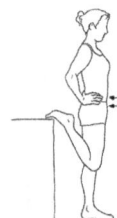

48. p133

Intermediate and advanced continued..

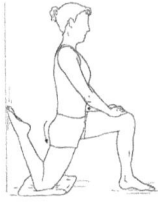 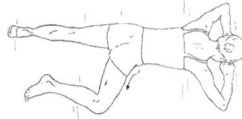

49. p133   **50.** p134

CHAPTER 8. Stretching and stability for the neck, shoulders and mid-back

Posture exercise and relaxing the neck and shoulder muscles

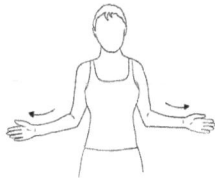 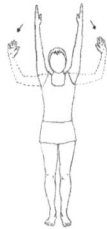 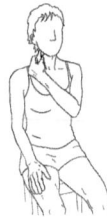 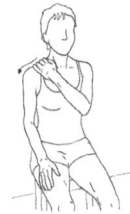

51. p143   **52.** p144   **53.** p145   **54.** p146

Neck stretches and stability

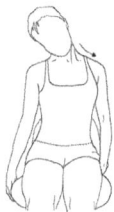 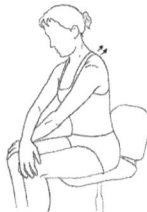 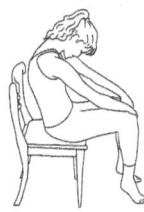 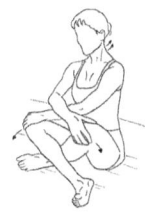

55. p146   **56.** p148   **57.** p148   **58.** p149

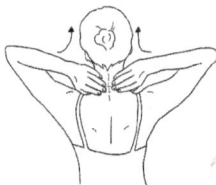 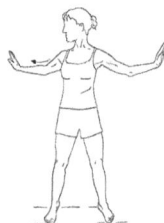 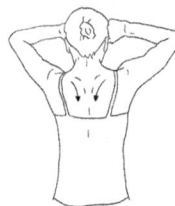 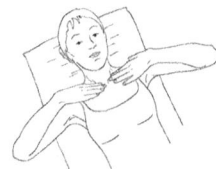

59. p150   **60.** p152   **61.** p152   **62.** p153

Mid back stretches and strengthening

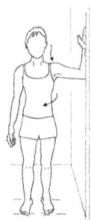

63. p155

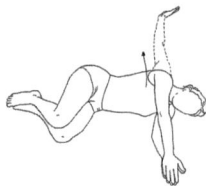

64. p156

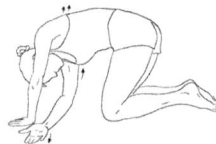

65. p156

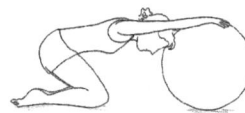

66. p157

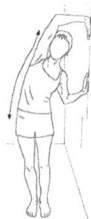

67. p157

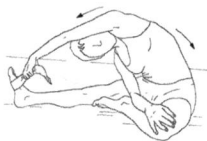

68. p158

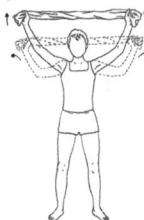

69. p158

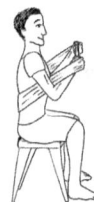

70. p159

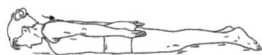

71. p159

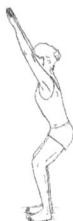

72. p160

CHAPTER 9. Posture - Exercises for postural types

Hyperkyphosis

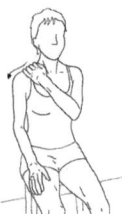

54. p146

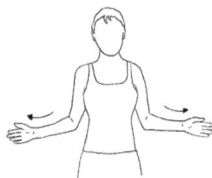

51. p143

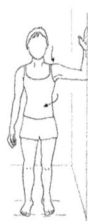

63. p155

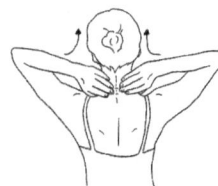

59. p150

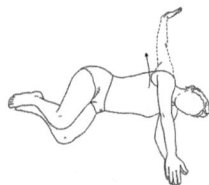

64. p156

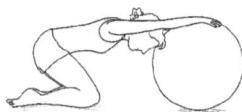

66. p157

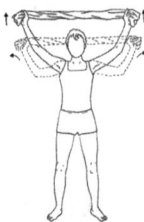

69. p158

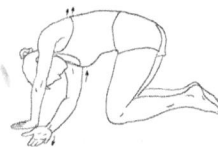

65. p156

Hyperkyphosis continued...

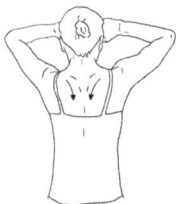

61. p152

Hyperlordosis

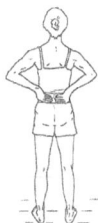

15. p98

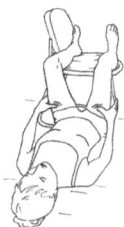

6. p56

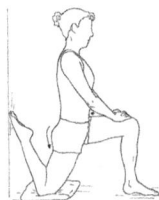

49. p133

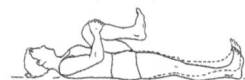

32. p117

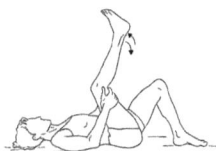

39. p125

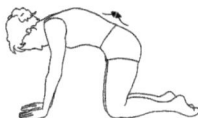

34. p118

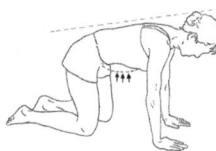

14. p97

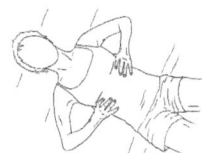

9. p94

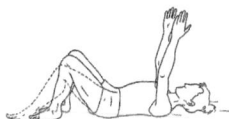

17&18. p99

Sway back

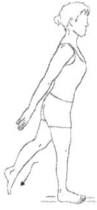

29. p109

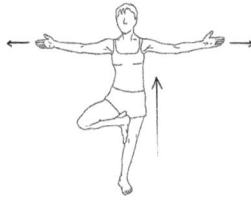

30. p109

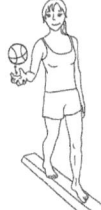

73. p237

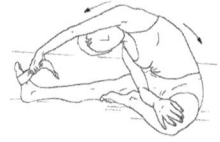

68. p158

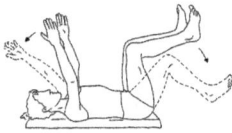

74. p239

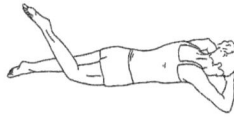

22. p102

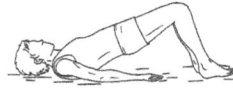

26. p107

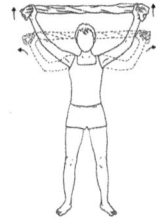

69. p158

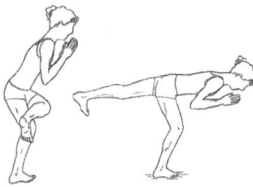

31. p110

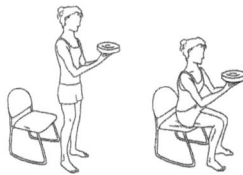

89. p251

Flat back

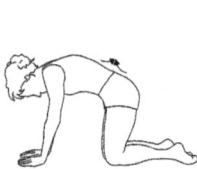

34. p118

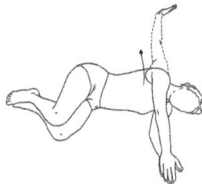

64. p156

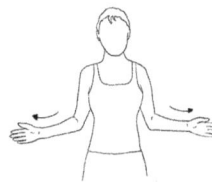

51. p143

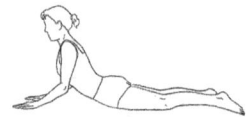

35. p118

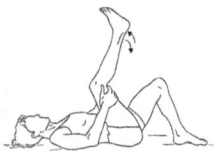

39. p125

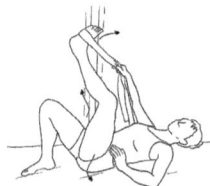

41. p127

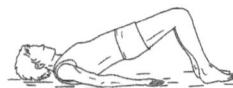

26. p107

Chapter 11. Advanced stability and strengthening with equipment

Using a foam beam

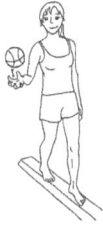

73. p237

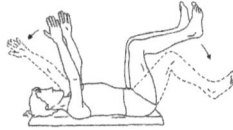

74. p239

Using a fitball

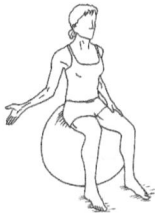

75. p239

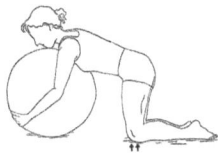

76. p240

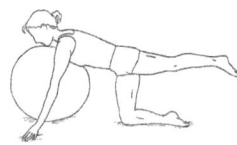

77. p240

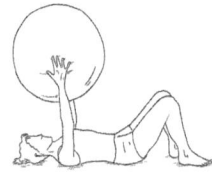

78. p240

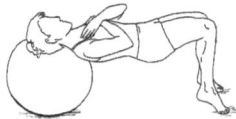

79. p241

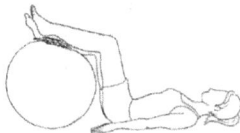

80. p242

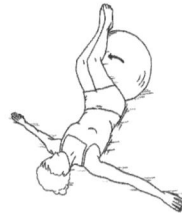

81. p242

Using an elasticised band

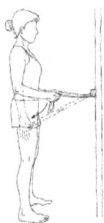

82. p243

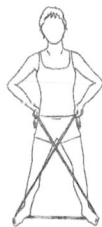

83. p243

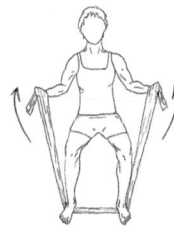

84. p244

Exercises to regain flexing confidence

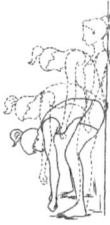

Rolling down the wall p247

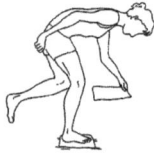

85. p248

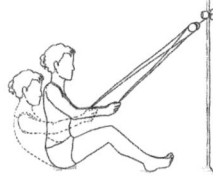

86. p249

Using weights

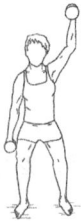

87. p250

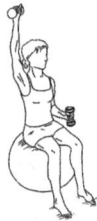

88. p250

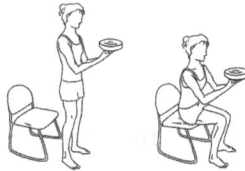

89. p251

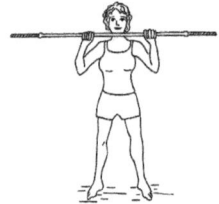

90. p251

APPENDIX III

FURTHER HELPFUL READING AND RESOURCES

It is not possible in a book of this length to go into great depth on the wide range of topics that are relevant to back pain. If you have further interest or questions in a specific area I highly recommend the following books.

READING

Pelvic floor

O'Dwyer, M, *Hold It Sister,* RedSok Publishing, Queensland, 2009

Chiarelli, P, *Women's Waterworks – Curing Incontinence,* Chiarelli Healthcare, Wallsend NSW, 2007

Wise, D, and Anderson, RA, *Headache in the Pelvis, 6th Edition: A New Understanding and Treatment for Chronic Pelvic Pain Syndromes,* National Center For Pelvic Pain, Occidental, California, 2007

Anatomy

Myers, TW, *Anatomy Trains,* Churchill Livingstone Elsevier, London, 2009

Nutrition and pain

Chadwick, V, *How to Live a Life without Pain,* Global Publishing Group, Victoria, 2013

Neural exercise

Butler, DS, *Mobilisation of the Nervous System,* Churchill Livingstone, London, 1991

Overcoming pain

Butler, DS, and Moseley, L, *Explain Pain,* Noi Group Publications, Australia, 2010

RESOURCES

3D Clinical Posture assessment

www.biocap.net

Overcoming Pain

www.greglehman.ca - Has an excellent booklet that can be used by clinicians and patients to address mind and body issues related to back pain. Also has podcasts on the topic of pain

www.noigroup.com - The Neuro Orthopaedic Institute offers a variety of courses, resources and publications on acute and chronic pain management

www.painscience.com - Explores common pain, treatment options, and tutorials. Useful search engine for the hundreds of articles that are referenced on the site

www.gradedmotorimagery.com - Brain-training exercises to assist with recovery and chronic pain management

www.bodymind.org - Evidence-based information on natural dietary supplements, nutrition and remedies for health of body and mind

www.bettermovement.org - Articles on the science of pain, posture, and movement. Considers how the brain and nervous system have more control than many people realise

www.bboyscience.com - Focuses on injury prevention and training, pain management, and recovery from injury

www.dermoneuromodulation.com - The connection between skin and nerves to change the experience of pain. Includes links on how the nervous system transmits pain signals

www.paintoolkit.org/resources/toolkits - Lists various resources including videos, an interactive section, and a downloadable easy-to-use guide on how to manage persistent pain

www.painmanagement.org.au - Provides support groups, phone help lines, monthly newsletters and tailored pain management plans

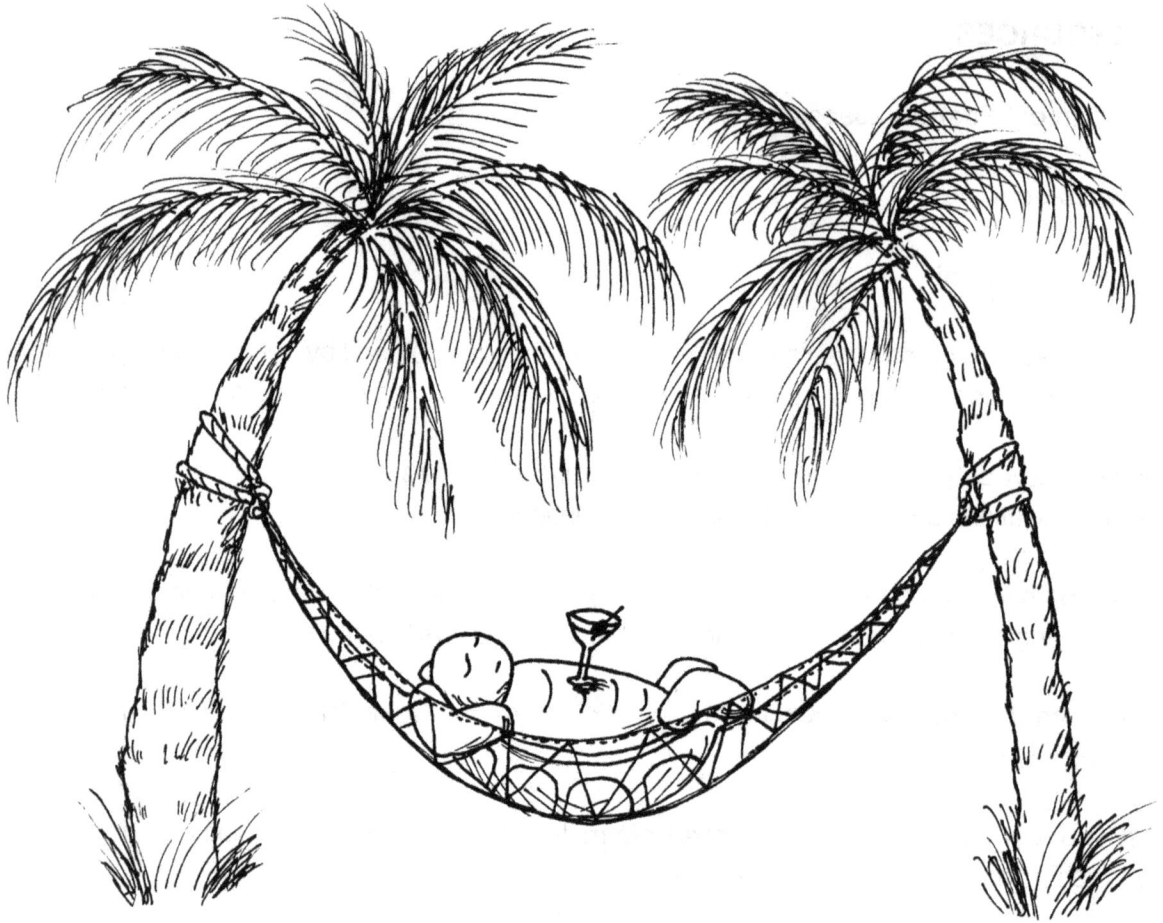

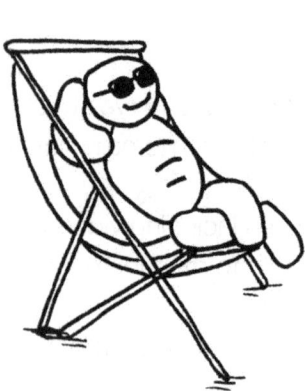

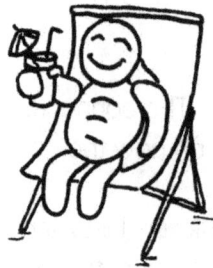

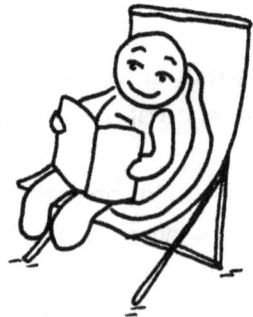

www.ingramcontent.com/pod-product-compliance
Lightning Source LLC
Chambersburg PA
CBHW081146270326
41930CB00014B/3051